The Patient's Guide to Fibromyalgia

By Matthew Dovie

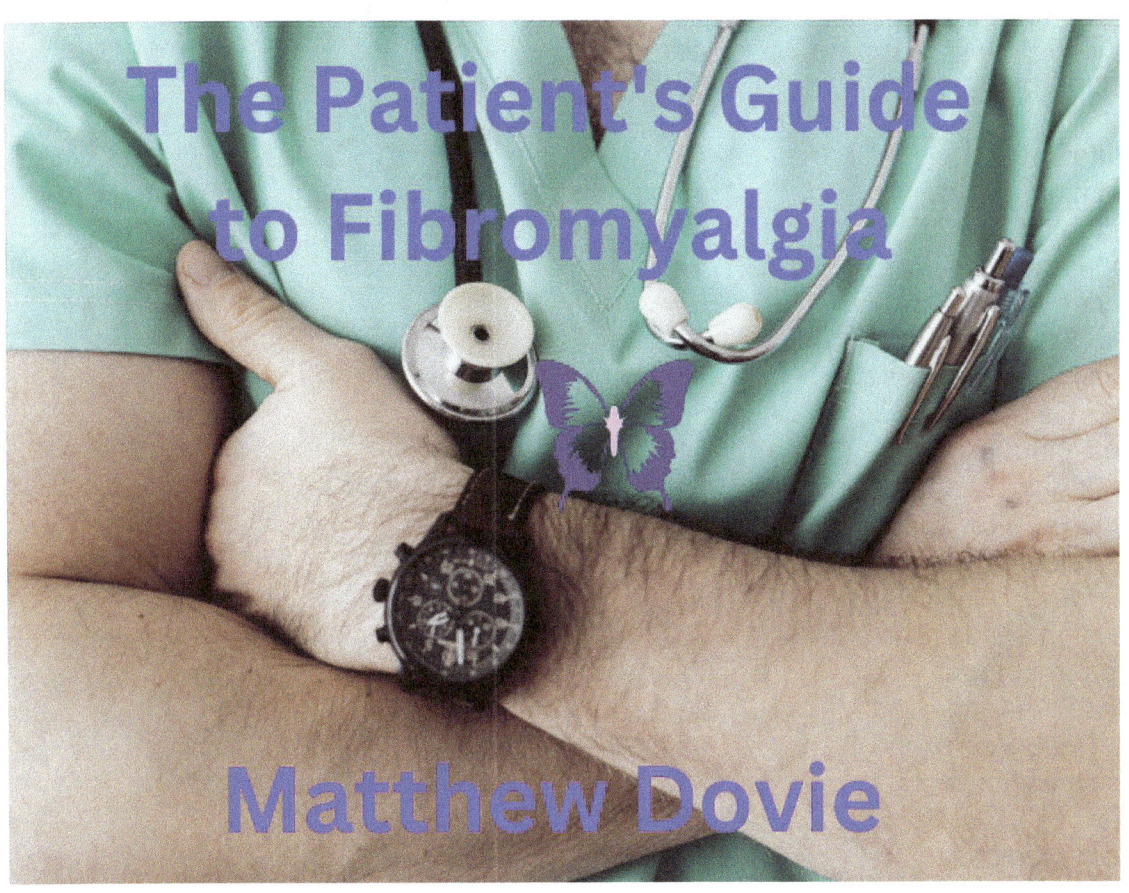

Table Of Contents

Introduction	3	SPG	110
The History of Fibromyalgia	9	TMJ	111
The Symptoms of Fibromyalgia	14	Sleep Treatments	114
Current Theories on FMS	18	Rheumatod Arthritis	117
The Canary in the Coal Mine	21	Lupus	120
Active Participant	24	OA	123
Become a Champion	25	Viscosupplementation	125
Find Your Team	27	PRP	126
Learn Patience	29	Endometriosis	127
Be Proactive	31	CBD & THC	129
Get Moving	33	Patient Advocacy	131
Social Support	35	Congratulations	135
Laughter	36	About the Author	136
Crank the Tunes	38		
Work on Sleep	39		
Rest	41		
Meditation	43		
Mindfulness	45		
Spirituality	47		
Food Intake	49		
Easy on the Carbs	51		
Avoid Fast Food	53		
Anxiety and Depression	56		
Fibromyalgia 101	59		
Sleep Study	61		
Attack Anxiety and Depression	64		
Vitamin Deficiencies	67		
The Value of Exercise	70		
Avoid Soda	73		
The Nightshade Plants	75		
Is Yeast a trigger?	77		
The 3 FDA Approved Meds	79		
Low Dose Naltrexone	83		
Muscle Relaxers	86		
TCA	89		
Opioid Medication	92		
Associated Conditions	95		
Chronic Fatigue Syndrome	98		
Migraine Headache	101		
CGRP	104		
Botox	107		

Introduction

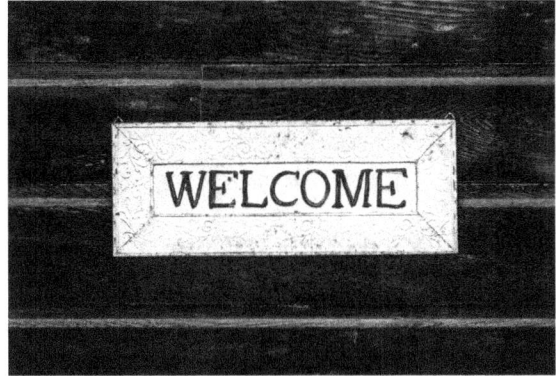

Welcome and congratulations as you have taken the first step to becoming an active participant in finding an effective treatment for your fibromyalgia pain!

It's an understatement to say that fibromyalgia is a complex and chronic pain disorder that affects millions of people worldwide. It is characterized by widespread musculoskeletal pain, fatigue, sleep disturbances, and cognitive impairments. Although fibromyalgia was recognized as a distinct condition relatively recently, it has gained increasing attention in the medical community over the past few decades. This introduction provides an overview of fibromyalgia, including its definition, prevalence, etiology, clinical presentation, impact on quality of life, diagnostic challenges, treatment approaches, and support strategies.

Fibromyalgia is a syndrome that is primarily characterized by chronic, widespread pain and tenderness in specific areas of the body, commonly referred to as tender points. In addition to pain, individuals with fibromyalgia often experience a range of symptoms, including fatigue, sleep disturbances, morning stiffness, headaches, irritable bowel syndrome, cognitive difficulties (often called "fibro fog"), and mood disturbances. The diagnosis of fibromyalgia is based on specific diagnostic criteria established by the American College of Rheumatology (ACR), which include a history of widespread pain lasting for at least three months and the presence of tenderness at 11 or more out of 18 specific tender points.

Fibromyalgia is a prevalent condition that affects approximately 2-8% of the general population. It is more common in women, with a female-to-male ratio ranging from 3:1 to 9:1. The condition can occur at any age, but it is most frequently diagnosed between the ages of 20 and 50. Fibromyalgia is also more prevalent in individuals with certain comorbid conditions, such as rheumatoid arthritis, systemic lupus erythematosus, and chronic fatigue syndrome.

The exact cause of fibromyalgia remains unknown, and it is likely multifactorial in nature. Research suggests that a combination of genetic, environmental, and psychological factors may contribute to its development. Some studies have identified genetic polymorphisms associated with fibromyalgia susceptibility, while others have found associations with physical trauma, infections, and psychosocial stressors. Furthermore, abnormalities in the central nervous system, including alterations in pain processing and neurotransmitter dysregulation, have been observed in individuals with fibromyalgia.

The clinical presentation of fibromyalgia is characterized by widespread pain and a variety of accompanying symptoms. The pain is typically described as a constant, dull ache that affects multiple areas of the body, including the muscles, joints, and soft tissues. It is often accompanied by fatigue, which can be severe and debilitating. Sleep disturbances, such as insomnia and non-restorative sleep, are also common and contribute to the overall fatigue experienced by individuals with fibromyalgia. Cognitive impairments, such as difficulties with memory, concentration, and attention, are frequently reported and can significantly impact daily functioning.

Fibromyalgia has a substantial impact on the quality of life of affected individuals. The chronic pain, fatigue, and associated symptoms can limit physical functioning, impair occupational performance, and interfere with social and leisure activities. The unpredictable nature of the condition, with symptoms fluctuating in severity, can make it challenging for individuals with fibromyalgia to plan and engage in regular activities. Furthermore, the invisible nature of the condition often leads to misunderstandings and skepticism from others, which can contribute to feelings of isolation and depression.

Diagnosing fibromyalgia can be challenging due to the subjective nature of the symptoms and the lack of specific diagnostic tests. The overlap of symptoms with other conditions, such as chronic fatigue syndrome and rheumatologic disorders, further complicates the diagnostic process. Additionally, the diagnostic criteria established by the ACR, while helpful, may not capture the full spectrum of fibromyalgia symptoms experienced by some individuals. As a result, there is often a delay in diagnosis, and many individuals with fibromyalgia may go through a long and frustrating journey to find answers and appropriate care.

The management of fibromyalgia typically involves a multidisciplinary approach that addresses both the physical and psychological aspects of the condition. There is no cure for fibromyalgia, but various treatment modalities aim to alleviate symptoms and improve overall functioning. Non-pharmacological interventions, such as exercise, physical therapy, cognitive-behavioral therapy, and stress management techniques, have been shown to be beneficial. Medications, including pain relievers, antidepressants, and anticonvulsants, may also be prescribed to help manage pain, improve sleep, and alleviate associated symptoms.

Living with fibromyalgia can be challenging, and individuals often require support to cope with the physical, emotional, and social impact of the condition. Support groups, both in-person and online, provide opportunities for individuals to connect with others who understand their experiences and share strategies for managing symptoms. Additionally, education about fibromyalgia, self-care techniques, and pacing activities can empower individuals to better manage their condition and improve their quality of life.

Research into fibromyalgia continues to expand our understanding of the condition and may lead to more targeted and effective treatments in the future. Advances in neuroimaging techniques, genetics, and the study of pain pathways are shedding light on the underlying mechanisms of fibromyalgia. Additionally, efforts to develop personalized medicine approaches and interventions that target specific symptom clusters hold promise for improving outcomes for individuals with fibromyalgia.

Fibromyalgia remains poorly understood, and its diagnosis and management present significant challenges. However, with a multidisciplinary approach that combines pharmacological and non-pharmacological interventions, along with support and coping strategies. My goal of this book is to give you a background on the history of fibromyalgia, theories about fibromyalgia and then the most current treatment options from both medications to lifestyle modifications to help you learn to better control your pain. Ongoing research and advancements in our understanding of fibromyalgia hold promise for better treatment options and improved outcomes in the future.

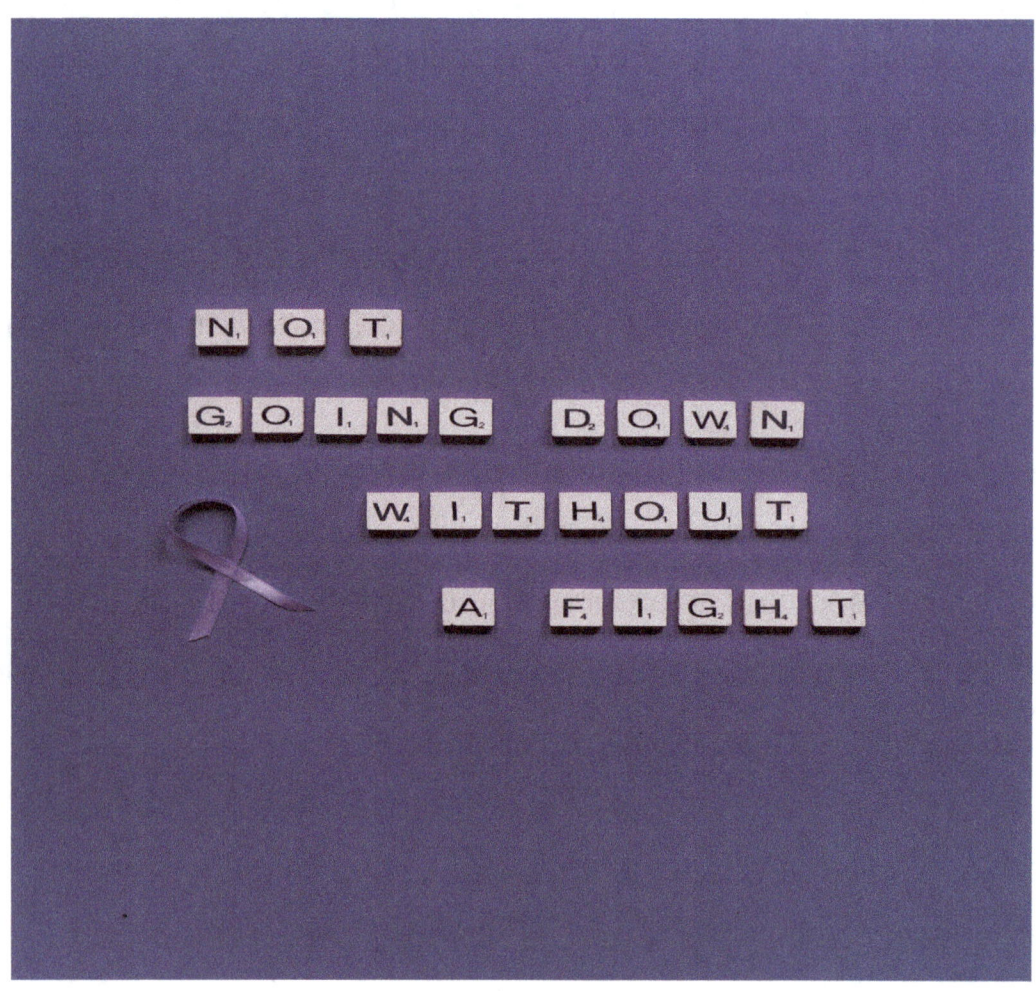

The History of Fibromyalgia

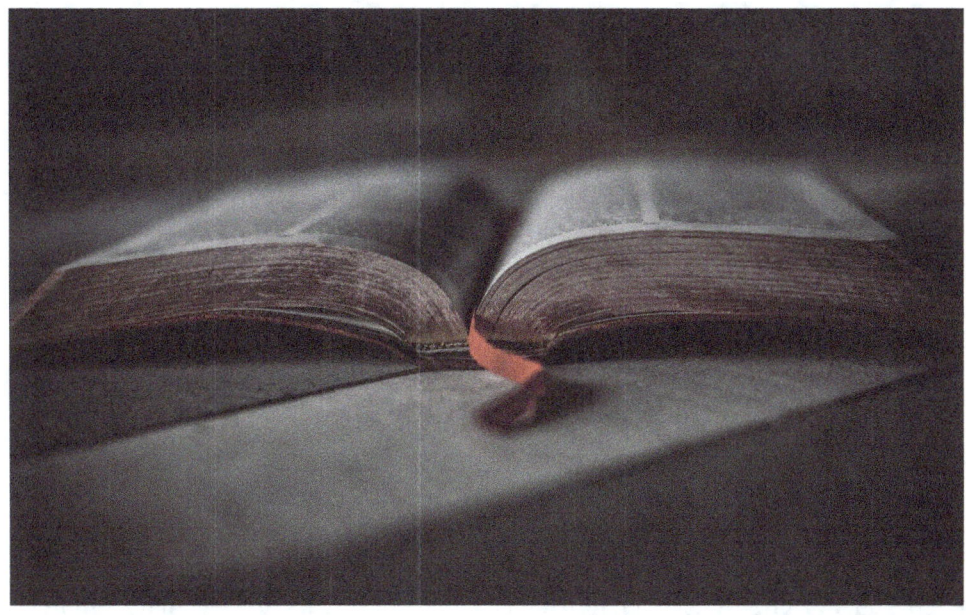

The history of fibromyalgia is relatively recent, with the condition being officially recognized and defined in the latter half of the 20th century. This section provides an overview of the key milestones and developments in the understanding of fibromyalgia, including its early descriptions, evolving diagnostic criteria, and the recognition of its impact on individuals' lives.

The origins of fibromyalgia can be traced back to the early medical literature, although it was not yet known by that name. Throughout history, descriptions of widespread pain and tender points can be found, often referred to as "rheumatism" or "neuralgia." However, it wasn't until the late 19th century that physicians began to observe and document a distinct set of symptoms that would later be associated with fibromyalgia.

One notable early description was made by Sir William Gowers in 1904, who identified a group of patients with generalized muscular rheumatism characterized by tender points and widespread pain. In the following decades, other physicians also made similar observations, including Smythe, Moldofsky, and Yunus, who laid the groundwork for the modern understanding of fibromyalgia.

The establishment of diagnostic criteria was crucial for recognizing fibromyalgia as a distinct condition. In 1981, Smythe and Moldofsky proposed a set of diagnostic criteria based on the presence of tender points and widespread pain. These criteria formed the foundation for subsequent developments in the field.

In 1990, the American College of Rheumatology (ACR) published the first official diagnostic criteria for fibromyalgia. These criteria required the presence of widespread pain in combination with tenderness at specific anatomical sites called tender points. According to these criteria, at least 11 out of 18 designated tender points had to be painful upon palpation for a diagnosis of fibromyalgia. The ACR criteria represented a significant step in standardizing the diagnosis of fibromyalgia and facilitating research in the field.

As awareness of fibromyalgia grew, it began to be recognized as a distinct syndrome with its own set of symptoms and characteristics. The term "fibromyalgia" itself was coined by Dr. Muhammad Yunus in 1981, deriving from the Latin words "fibro" (fibrous tissue), "myo" (muscles), and "algia" (pain). This name reflected the widespread pain and tender points associated with the condition.

Over time, the understanding of fibromyalgia expanded beyond its physical manifestations. It became evident that individuals with fibromyalgia also experienced a range of other symptoms, including fatigue, sleep disturbances, cognitive impairments, and mood disorders. This recognition helped shift the focus from purely musculoskeletal aspects to a more comprehensive understanding of fibromyalgia as a multi-systemic disorder.

As the recognition of fibromyalgia grew, so did research efforts to understand its underlying mechanisms and develop effective treatments. Advances in medical imaging techniques, such as positron emission tomography (PET) and functional magnetic resonance imaging (fMRI), have provided insights into the central nervous system abnormalities associated with fibromyalgia, including altered pain processing and neurotransmitter dysregulation.

Additionally, genetic studies have identified potential genetic predispositions to fibromyalgia, highlighting the complex interplay between genetic and environmental factors in its development. These advancements have deepened our understanding of fibromyalgia as a neurobiological condition rather than a purely psychogenic disorder, dispelling previous misconceptions.

Fibromyalgia has a significant impact on the lives of individuals affected by the condition. The recognition of fibromyalgia as a legitimate and disabling condition has led to increased advocacy efforts and support networks. Patient advocacy groups and organizations have played a vital role in raising awareness, promoting research, and providing resources for individuals with fibromyalgia.

The increased recognition of fibromyalgia as a chronic pain condition has also contributed to improvements in healthcare delivery and treatment options. Multidisciplinary approaches, including a combination of pharmacological and non-pharmacological interventions, are now recognized as the standard of care for fibromyalgia management.

The history of fibromyalgia reflects the evolving understanding and recognition of the condition as a distinct syndrome. From its early descriptions as "rheumatism" to the establishment of diagnostic criteria and the recognition of its impact on individuals' lives, fibromyalgia has undergone significant milestones. Continued research efforts and advocacy work have deepened our understanding of fibromyalgia's underlying mechanisms and improved treatment options, leading to better support for individuals living with this complex chronic pain condition.

The Symptoms of Fibromyalgia

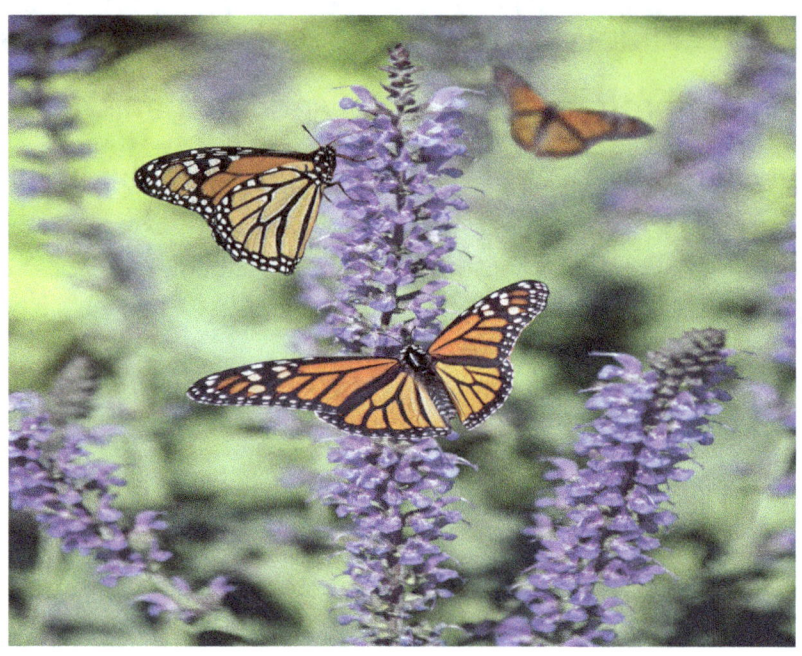

While the symptoms can vary from person to person, there are several common symptoms that are frequently reported by individuals with fibromyalgia. This section provides an in-depth exploration of the most prevalent symptoms associated with fibromyalgia, including pain, fatigue, sleep disturbances, cognitive impairments, and mood disorders.

Widespread pain is the hallmark symptom of fibromyalgia. Individuals with fibromyalgia experience chronic pain that is widespread and affects multiple areas of the body. The pain is often described as a constant, dull ache that can be accompanied by tenderness at specific anatomical sites known as tender points. These tender points are typically located in areas such as the neck, shoulders, chest, hips, and knees. The pain may also migrate to different areas of the body over time. The intensity of the pain can vary, and it may be exacerbated by physical activity, stress, or changes in weather.

Fatigue is another common symptom experienced by individuals with fibromyalgia. It is not simply a feeling of tiredness but rather a pervasive sense of exhaustion that is not alleviated by rest or sleep. The fatigue associated with fibromyalgia can be debilitating and significantly impact daily functioning. It may manifest as a general lack of energy, difficulty initiating or sustaining physical activities, and a feeling of mental and physical heaviness. Fatigue can also contribute to cognitive impairments, commonly referred to as "fibro fog," which will be discussed in more detail later.

Sleep disturbances are prevalent among individuals with fibromyalgia. Despite feeling fatigued, many individuals with fibromyalgia experience difficulties falling asleep and staying asleep throughout the night. Sleep disturbances in fibromyalgia can manifest as insomnia, characterized by difficulty falling asleep or maintaining sleep, as well as non-restorative sleep, where individuals do not wake up feeling refreshed. Sleep disruptions may be due to pain, restless leg syndrome, or other sleep disorders commonly associated with fibromyalgia. The lack of restful sleep can further exacerbate fatigue and contribute to overall symptoms.

Cognitive impairments, often referred to as "fibro fog," are commonly reported by individuals with fibromyalgia. These cognitive difficulties can affect various aspects of mental functioning, including memory, concentration, attention, and information processing speed. Individuals with fibromyalgia may experience difficulties remembering details, multitasking, finding words, and staying focused on tasks. The cognitive impairments can have a significant impact on daily activities, work performance, and overall quality of life. While the exact cause of fibro fog is not fully understood, it is believed to be related to the underlying neurobiological changes associated with fibromyalgia.

Mood disorders, such as depression and anxiety, are frequently comorbid with fibromyalgia. The chronic pain, fatigue, and other symptoms associated with fibromyalgia can take a toll on an individual's emotional well-being. Feelings of frustration, irritability, and sadness are common among individuals with fibromyalgia. Depression and anxiety can further exacerbate the perception of pain and contribute to the overall burden of the condition. Treating mood disorders in conjunction with managing the physical symptoms of fibromyalgia is essential for a comprehensive approach to fibromyalgia management.

The most common symptoms of fibromyalgia include widespread pain, fatigue, sleep disturbances, cognitive impairments (fibro fog), and mood disorders. These symptoms can significantly impact an individual's quality of life, making it crucial to address and manage them as part of a multidisciplinary treatment approach. While there is no cure for fibromyalgia, various interventions, including medication, exercise, stress management, and cognitive-behavioral therapy, can help alleviate symptoms and improve overall well-being. A comprehensive understanding of the most common symptoms of fibromyalgia is essential for healthcare professionals and individuals affected by the condition to effectively manage its impact.

Current Theories of Fibromyalgia

Current theories on fibromyalgia aim to shed light on the underlying mechanisms and factors contributing to the development and persistence of thecondition. While the exact cause of fibromyalgia remains unknown, several theories have emerged based on research findings and clinical observations. This section provides an overview of some of the current theories on fibromyalgia, including central sensitization, neuroendocrine abnormalities, genetic factors, and psychological factors.

One of the leading theories on fibromyalgia is central sensitization. According to this theory, individuals with fibromyalgia have an abnormality in the central nervous system's pain processing mechanisms. It is believed that there is an amplification of pain signals in the brain, leading to an exaggerated pain response to both painful and non-painful stimuli. This hypersensitivity to pain can explain the widespread pain experienced by individuals with fibromyalgia, as well as the tenderness at specific tender points.

Research has shown that individuals with fibromyalgia have alterations in the levels of neurotransmitters, such as serotonin, dopamine, and glutamate, which play a role in pain processing. Additionally, functional neuroimaging studies have demonstrated abnormal activity in pain-related brain regions, further supporting the central sensitization theory.

Another theory proposes that neuroendocrine abnormalities contribute to the development of fibromyalgia. Neuroendocrine abnormalities involve dysregulation of hormones and neurotransmitters that are involved in pain modulation, sleep regulation, and stress response. Research suggests that individuals with fibromyalgia may have altered levels of neurotransmitters, such as serotonin, norepinephrine, and substance P, which can affect pain perception and mood regulation.

Additionally, abnormalities in the hypothalamic-pituitary-adrenal (HPA) axis, which is responsible for regulating the body's response to stress, have been observed in individuals with fibromyalgia. Dysregulation of cortisol, the primary stress hormone, and abnormalities in the release of other hormones, such as growth hormone and thyroid hormone, have been reported. These neuroendocrine abnormalities may contribute to the symptoms of fibromyalgia, including pain, fatigue, and sleep disturbances.

There is growing evidence supporting a genetic component in the development of fibromyalgia. Family and twin studies have suggested a higher prevalence of fibromyalgia among first-degree relatives, indicating a potential genetic predisposition. Several candidate genes have been identified as potential contributors to fibromyalgia susceptibility, including genes involved in neurotransmitter regulation, pain perception, and the immune system.

However, the genetic factors associated with fibromyalgia are likely complex, involving multiple genes and gene-environment interactions.

Further research is needed to unravel the specific genetic mechanisms underlying fibromyalgia and their role in the condition's pathogenesis.

Psychological factors, such as stress, trauma, and mood disorders, are believed to play a role in the development and exacerbation of fibromyalgia symptoms. It is well-established that individuals with fibromyalgia often experience high levels of psychological distress, including depression and anxiety. These psychological factors can influence pain perception and amplify the impact of fibromyalgia on an individual's well-being.

Stress, both acute and chronic, has been associated with the onset and worsening of fibromyalgia symptoms. The physiological response to stress, including the release of stress hormones, can exacerbate central sensitization and contribute to the amplification of pain signals. Furthermore, traumatic experiences, such as physical or emotional abuse, have been identified as potential risk factors for developing fibromyalgia.

Current theories on fibromyalgia suggest that a combination of factors, including central sensitization, neuroendocrine abnormalities, genetic predisposition, and psychological factors, contribute to the development and persistence of the condition. These theories provide insights into the complex nature of fibromyalgia and highlight the need for a multidimensional approach to its diagnosis and management.

The Canary in the Coal Mine

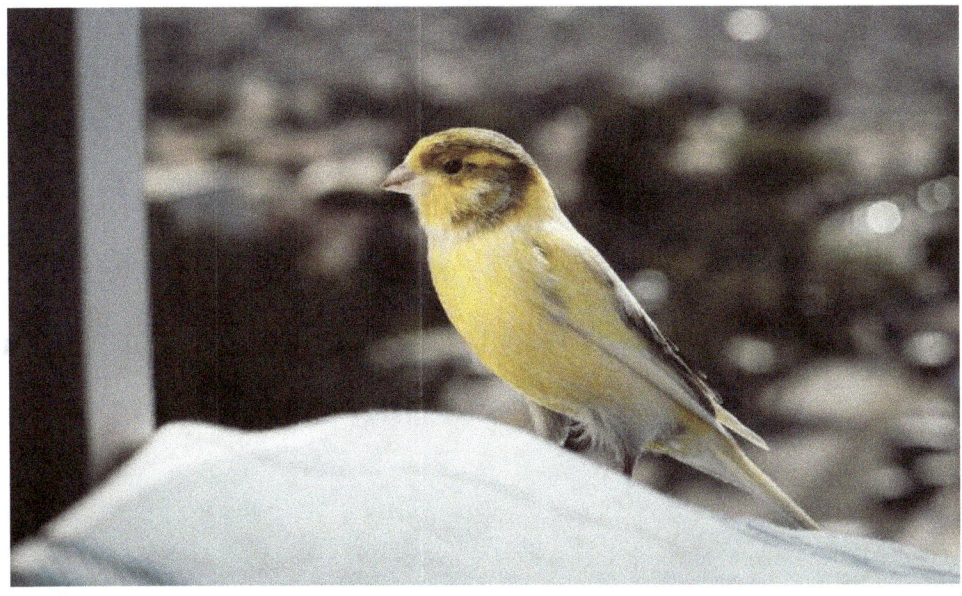

The theory of the canary in the coal mine draws an analogy between the condition of fibromyalgia and the role of canaries in early warning systems for detecting harmful gases in coal mines. This theory suggests that fibromyalgia may serve as a warning sign or indicator of broader systemic dysfunction in the body. This section explores the theory of the canary in the coal mine in the context of fibromyalgia, highlighting the potential implications for understanding the condition and its relationship to overall health.

In coal mining, canaries were used as a vital early warning system to detect the presence of toxic gases, particularly carbon monoxide and methane. These gases, if undetected, could lead to asphyxiation or explosions. Canaries were highly sensitive to the toxic gases, and if they showed signs of distress or illness, it signaled the need for immediate evacuation of the mine.

The theory of the canary in the coal mine draws on this historical context to suggest that fibromyalgia may similarly serve as a sentinel, indicating a broader dysfunction or imbalance within the body. It proposes that the symptoms experienced by individuals with fibromyalgia may reflect an underlying systemic disturbance, with fibromyalgia being a visible manifestation of a more complex and interconnected health picture.

Fibromyalgia is characterized by widespread pain, fatigue, sleep disturbances, cognitive impairments, and other symptoms that can affect various bodily systems. While the exact cause of fibromyalgia is unknown, the theory of the canary in the coal mine suggests that fibromyalgia may be a result of dysregulation or dysfunction in multiple systems, including the central nervous system, neuroendocrine system, immune system, and psychological factors.

Research has shown that individuals with fibromyalgia often exhibit alterations in pain processing, neurotransmitter imbalances, abnormalities in stress response systems (such as the hypothalamic-pituitary-adrenal axis), and immune system dysregulation. These findings support the idea that fibromyalgia involves complex interactions among various physiological systems, contributing to the development and persistence of the condition.

Moreover, studies have demonstrated that individuals with fibromyalgia often experience comorbidities such as irritable bowel syndrome, migraines, temporomandibular joint disorder, and mood disorders like depression and anxiety. These comorbidities further support the theory of fibromyalgia as a canary, indicating broader systemic dysfunction that extends beyond musculoskeletal pain.

Viewing fibromyalgia through the lens of the canary in the coal mine has important implications for the diagnosis and treatment of the condition. Recognizing fibromyalgia as a potential indicator of underlying systemic dysfunction prompts healthcare providers to take a holistic and comprehensive approach to evaluation and treatment.

Diagnosis should involve a thorough assessment of an individual's symptoms, medical history, and potential comorbidities. It is important to consider the interconnectedness of physiological systems and to address not only the symptoms but also the underlying contributing factors.

The theory of the canary in the coal mine provides a valuable perspective on fibromyalgia, suggesting that the condition may serve as an indicator of broader systemic dysfunction.

Active Participant

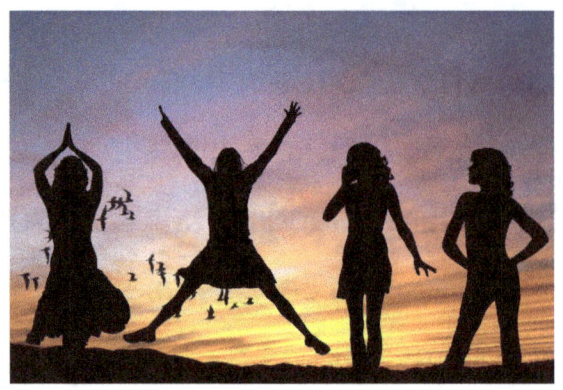

It is important for all patients with fibromyalgia to be involved as an active participant in their treatment plan. This seems obvious but too many patients take a passive approach to their healing and care.

Too many times I have treated patients who don't follow the recommendations and plans given to them and then are surprised when they haven't made any progress. As you know, treating pain is complex. You must treat both the physical, emotional, psychological and spiritual nature of one's being to find long term benefit. There are no shortcuts and no magic pill that will take all the pain away.

By reading this book you are taking a good first step to becoming an active participant in your care. My goal is to show you ways to become further involved as an active participant including nutrition, exercise, meditation, medication and exciting interventional pain treatments.

I'm excited you have decided to join me on this journey.

Become a Champion

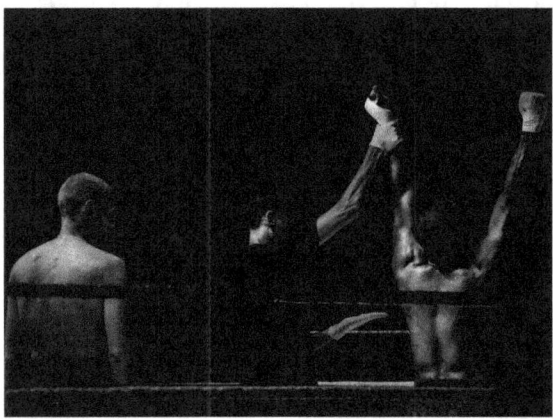

To effectively treat your fibromyalgia pain you must learn to become a champion. A champion is defined as an individual who overcomes great odds to achieve their goals.

This is an active approach to taking back your life. The first step is to pick one activity that you had quit due to you pain. This can be as simple as walking up the hill to the mailbox or going to the grocery store. There is no quit in a champion, you will start by telling your pain "I'm taking this back!". As you start to slowly add back more activities you will gain more confidence and improve your quality of life. These small victories will improve your mood and outlook. Just like any champion, the road to success will have its highs and lows. Don't become frustrated if you have a setback, only by failing can we learn to succeed.

By winning more and more of these small victories you will learn to control your pain and not let your pain control you. When you learn that you control your pain you will become a champion!

Find Your Team

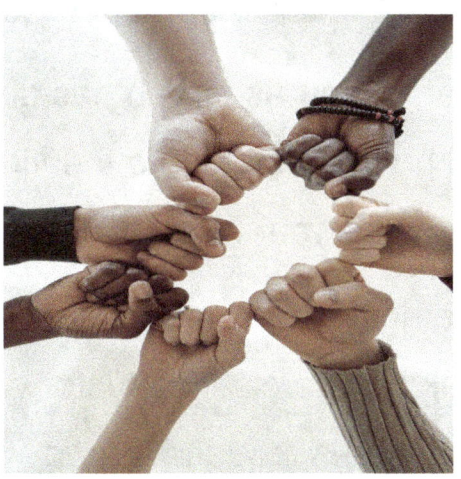

To treat your fibromyalgia you will need to actively seek a health care team dedicated to achieving your goals. I hope to weaponize you with actionable information to help you begin this journey. You will want to seek providers that take a multidimensional approach. Ideally you will have a healthcare provider who can help you manage any issues needed. Find a provider that doesn't treat you like cattle. Find a provider that takes the time to know their patients and not someone who kicks you out the door after 10 minutes. Avoid the 'pill mill' clinics! If you suffer with underlying anxiety and depression, which is almost every patient, you will want to also work with a pain psychologist or psychiatrist to help with coping skills.

Some additional treatments that I recommend would involve joining a a pain support group, either one specifically for fibromyalgia or one for chronic pain. Having a support group to vent at, share ideas, share victories or frustrations is a critical component to healing.

I like to call it the "Oprah effect" as Oprah has done wonders with addressing issues and bringing them into the viewer's living room. So can these support groups be your "Oprah effect".

As you become a more active participant, I then encourage my patients to actively seek an exercise instructor with experience in pain patients. Yoga, Tai Chi, Pilates, aquatic therapy are all wonderful examples of improving strength and flexibility while decreasing pain.

The goal is finding the right members to fill out your pain fighting team!

Learn Patience

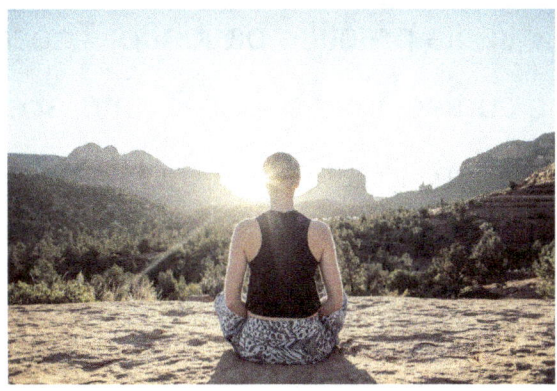

To treat your fibromyalgia, a patient must learn patience. Your chronic pain is a complex web that developed through a course of unfortunate events and set up an ingrained neurological pathway signal of pain to your brain. I give the example of a girl walking across a dewy meadow. A girl walks across the meadow in the morning, you would not see her path later in the day. However, if that same girl walks across the meadow everyday for the next 6 months, even if she then misses one day you will be able to see the path she has walked. This is the same as chronic pain patterns.

It took a long time to get to the point of your chronic pain and your treatment will also take a period of time and be a process to heal.

Don't expect any magical healthcare provider to be able to solve all your problems in one visit.

Instead, understand that a patient with patience and understanding will have the best results. Patience also helps to curb anxiety that intensifies pain and hinders the healing process.

I recommend mindful meditation, prayer, exercise or relaxation techniques to help patients practice patience. These techniques will help decrease stress cortisol levels, boost natural endorphins and will help patients become more in tune with their body and help the healing process.

Be Proactive

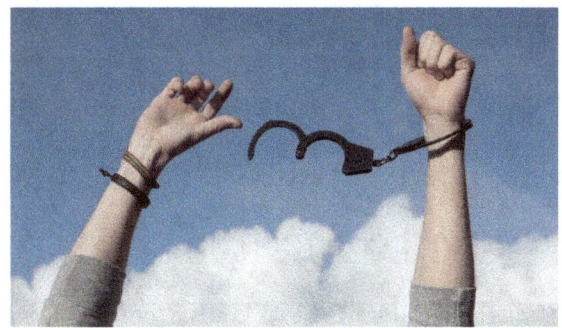

Although this was stated above, it is worth repeating and describing further. To help find an effective treatment for you fibromyalgia, I require my patients to become proactive. This requires patients to take the initiative to improve their situation. Instead of letting your current circumstances be the driving force of determining your future I help patients to determine their choices and act to improve their situation instead of only reacting.

I help my patients realize that even when they feel they have limited choices or little hope there is always a direction that allows a patient to be in control of their pain and therefore their outcome. I teach my patients that they get to choose how their pain and conditions define them. Patients that currently feel helpless are allowing their circumstances and conditions to control them. For example, a helpless patient may respond with "there's nothing I can do about my pain". I teach my patients to focus their time and energy on things they have control over. For example, my patients get to decide if they will wake up and do something productive today. They get to decide if they will interact positively with their family despite how their pain is making them feel. I help to teach my patients ways to empower their situation. That feeling of empowerment propels patients to gain more and more control of their pain. Focusing on items we do control instead of the items we can't control help to reduce stress levels which decrease anxiety and help my patients to better cope with their pain.

I teach patients to eliminate certain phrases including: "I can't", "I must", "If only", 'there's nothing I can do". I help patients break the handcuffs of negativity that surround and influence their painful condition. I help patients look at alternatives so that they can instead take a different approach and be in control, only then can you find an effective treatment plan for your fibromyalgia.

Get Moving!

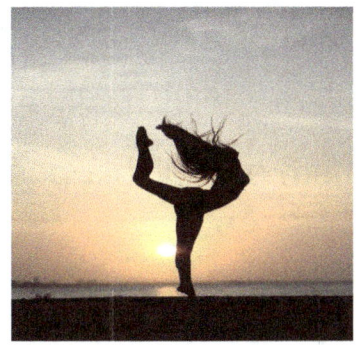

To effectively treat your fibromyalgia, all patients need some level of an exercise routine. Obviously, many pain conditions can significantly limit the types of exercise a patient can perform but every patient can do some level activity above their sedentary status.

The gold standard exercise for chronic back pain patients is aquatic therapy. In fact, most patients seem to respond to aquatic therapy as it is a way to improve range of motion, flexibility, and attain some level of cardiovascular workout in a controlled environment that is less stressful to the joints than land based activities.

Low impact yoga or some form of a daily stretching routine is another excellent form of daily exercise that almost all patients should add to their daily routine. Fibromyalgia patients seem to be a particular set of patients that I have personally witnessed make great strides.
For wheelchair bound patients, there are now excellent chair based exercise classes. In my 23 years of practice I've literally never found a patient that couldn't benefit from some type of exercise routine.

A daily exercise routine, improves strength and flexibility which can help patients avoid falls. Falls are very common with pain patients and can lead to further pain and disability. Daily exercise will improve a patient's mood and help them establish a positive routine to their day.

Check with your health care provider before starting an exercise routine. Afterwards, find some movement that you can stick with and perform most days of the week and get moving!

Social Support

An often overlooked part of any patient's treatment plan is a friend to offer support. A friend, or some form of a supportive social network, is key to any recovery. This can range from a family member, an understanding neighbor, friend or online support group.

It's seems that for some of my pain patients I act as much a counselor rather than a traditional medical provider. Sometimes patients just simply need someone to vent their frustrations and aggravations to, someone who will take the time to listen and empathize with their situation. For some of my patients, a trip to the office is the highlight of their social calendar for the month.

I encourage all patients to find someone who they can spend quality time with in a supportive and caring manner. This social bond has an effective psychological impact on a patient's recovery. Having social support helps to motivate patients to be more active and involved. For some patients, their social network is severely limited due to their disability or lack of proximity to family and friends. Even patients with severe isolation issues can find some form of social network. I encourage home bound patients to join an online therapy or support group that is tailored to patients with their similar condition. This can be an effective tool to use as a sounding board for advice or support.

Laughter

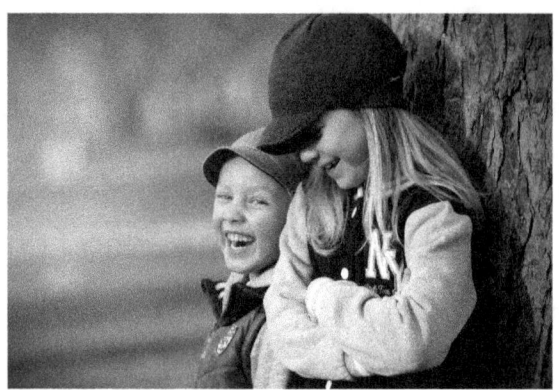

A very successful and overlooked tool in the treatment of chronic pain is laughter. Laughter holds many known benefits for the body from both a psychological and physiological perspective.

Laughter is known to lower blood pressure and reduce stress hormone levels. Laughter, the actual act of laughing, can also improve cardiac health. Laughter is known to improve immune function which is a vital factor in your recovery. Laughing also triggers the release of endorphins which are your body's natural pain killers. Laughing also improves a patient's general well being. Laughter improves circulation and smooth muscle relaxation, of vital importance to patient's suffering from chronic muscular pain conditions and ailments.

Beyond these physical responses to laughter, I have found that patients who regularly incorporate laughter have an improved outlook to their pain. Patient's who have the insight to laugh at their circumstances have improved quality of life and improved overall function. The old theory of the glass half full really does seem to apply to pain patients and helps to set realistic expectations.

So find a few moments every day to add some laughter back into your life.

Crank up the Tunes!

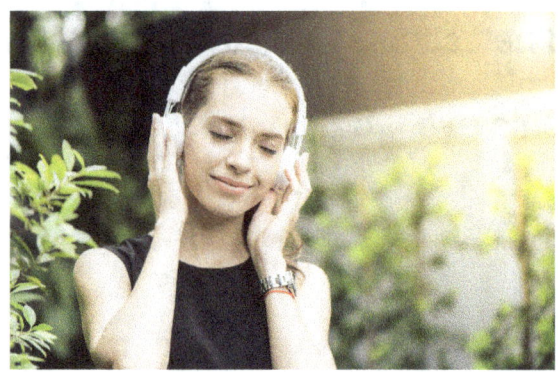

Music has the ability to be an amazing adjunctive therapy to help treat chronic pain. Neuroscientists have discovered that listening to music heightens positive emotion through stimulating dopamine levels. Dopamine has powerful effects on the reward center in the brain that affect emotion and pain control. Dopamine release from music has also been tied to improving motivation which helps gives pain patients the energy to be more active. Numerous studies have shown that athletes who train with music have improved endurance.

Music helps manage and control pain in a multitude of factors. Music has the ability to reduce stress and anxiety. Research shows music can prevent anxiety-induced increases in heart rate and high blood pressure. Listening to music can help reduce cortisol levels, a stress hormone. The power of music seems to act on both a physiological as well as psychological level to help patients better manage their pain. Music therapy is now being used as a means of conditioning patients to relax and release pain and stress.

Work on your Sleep

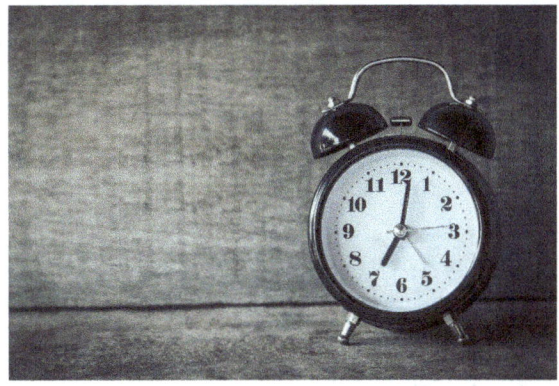

One common thread for the majority of fibromyalgia patients is poor sleep. Yes, pain can keep patients from a good night sleep, but more and more studies are revealing that many pain conditions, specifically chronic pain conditions like Fibromyalgia are worsened by poor sleep patterns. Altered sleep patterns or poor sleep will impact the neurological, psychological, and physical function of the body. It has the same affect as a battery that never fully recharges.

I order sleep studies on all of my chronic pain patients. Many patients falsely believe that sleep studies are only valuable if a patient snores or has sleep apnea but this is false. Many patients have an underlying condition that has not been addressed. Sleep apnea can range from a true obstruction but can also pertain to patients that hold their breath while they sleep, so although they don't have a classic snore they still have poor perfusion of oxygen to the organs and this can directly impact the body's own healing mechanisms. Sleep studies can also identify what stages of sleep a patient is in the majority of the night.

Most chronic pain patients and classically Fibromyalgia patients spend the majority of their night in lighter stages of sleep and never enter the deeper restorative phases. Impaired sleep can also exacerbate other chronic health conditions including Hypertension and Type 2 Diabetes.

A first step toward helping to treat your chronic pain is to rule out or treat any underlying sleep disturbances.

In later chapters I will discuss some effective medication and interventions to improve sleep.

Rest

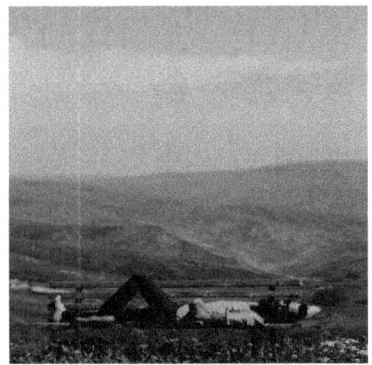

To help effectively treat your fibromyalgia you must become more active and vigilant in your own recovery and yes this also applies to taking advantage of your rest. Rest come in many forms from improving your sleep, which we have already discussed, naps, meditation, stretching, and an approach to activity known as a active rest.

So much of our life seems to be some automated loop, whether that is our routine of running off to work in the morning or running our kids to school and various activities. People adapt to their hectic loop of a life by running from one activity to the next, pumping caffeine into their bodies at the local java hut to keep moving.

There is an argument that hitting the pause button and trying to find a better balance to our hectic lives and finding opportunities to rest is an excellent way to heal our body and our soul. A conscious approach to adding active rest based activities is a natural approach to living within your bodies circadian rhythm. Most research show that humans are designed to take an afternoon nap. Although a nap is not possible for most, finding 10 minutes to meditate or take a nature stroll seems to do wonders. For patients able to exercise, I recommend alternating between a heavy exercise day with a lighter exercise day to not over stress our body. For patients with more disabilities to activity, I recommend trying to stagger doctor appointments or busy days so as to not overwhelm yourself psychologically or physically.

I am not promoting a couch potato lifestyle rather I'm simply recognizing that making a conscious decision to rest on the couch and read a book or relax the mind periodically is a healthy choice.

Meditation

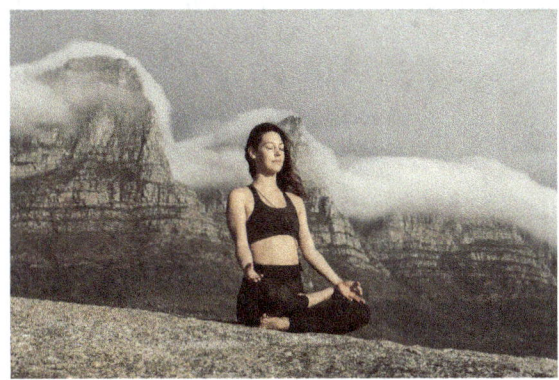

Meditation is an effective tool to help avoid additional prescription medications and help cure pain. Meditation can rewire the brain's pain circuitry. Neuronal pathways within the brain get programmed every time you expect pain to occur. In time, less and less stimulus is needed to trigger the pain reflex. Eventually, the simple thought of pain becomes the true source, not necessarily the ailment itself.

Meditation can unhook your emotional reaction to pain. My patients can get stuck in a brutal feedback loop, without even realizing it. Their anticipation of pain creates stress, stress leads to physical tension within the body — especially near the painful area which ultimately leads to more pain.

Meditation teaches you how to emotionally detach from your negative thoughts and physical sensations, where you no longer expect pain, nor resist it when it does occur.

Meditation can also help us treat our natural flight or fight response to pain which can be abnormally triggered in chronic pain patients. The flight or fight increases cortisol stress levels. Elevated stress levels increase blood pressure, increase inflammatory markers and increase pain. Meditation helps to reduce these harmful stress hormone levels.

Meditation can also boost natural endorphin levels which act as a natural pain reliever, decrease cortisol levels and allow patients to be in control of their pain.

Mindfulness

For motivated patients I encourage them to study and incorporate mindfulness into their daily routine. Mindfulness is the psychological process off bringing one's attention to experiences in the moment. It is best accomplished with training and the practice of meditation. Mindfulness interventions are effective in reducing rumination and worry. Rumination on one's pain or illness exacerbates depression and underlying anxiety conditions. A classic example is with my Fibromyalgia patients, they commonly ruminate on the condition and identify themselves as 'Fibro' instead of focusing on a more positive aspect of their life.

Classic mindfulness treatments I recommend to patients include a very basic mindfulness meditation where a patient sits and quietly focuses on their natural breathing. The patients are taught to allow thoughts to come and go without any judgement, simply allow the thoughts to dissolve away and then focus back on their breathing. A simple 3-5 minutes per day will start to show dramatic benefits in as little as 2 weeks as patients learn to wipe away anxiety and help to distract from the negative effects of pain on the mind.

A few apps that I have found helpful for patients to practice mindfulness include: Headspace, Aura and the app Stop Breath & Think.

As a patient incorporates a mindfulness approach to their daily routine, pain levels decrease, anxiety decreases, empowerment increases and patients inch closer to a more effective treatment for their pain.

Spirituality

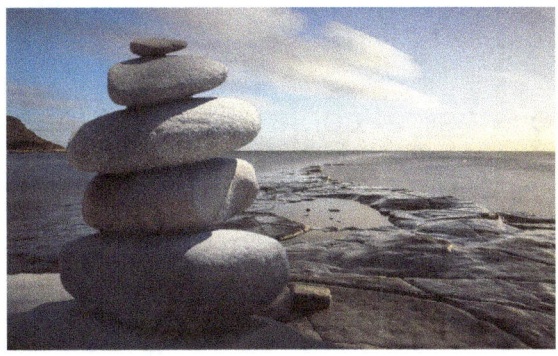

Fibromyalgia is a misunderstood and complex condition to treat. Research on the biology and neurobiology of pain has shown a relationship between spirituality and pain. Using a number of cognitive and behavioral strategies to cope with pain, including religious/spiritual factors, such as prayer or seeking spiritual support to manage pain is an essential component to finding an effective treatment for your pain.

Many patients confuse spirituality with religion. Although the two can overlap there is a difference between religion and spirituality. Religion is an organized faith system grounded in institutional practices while spirituality is grounded in personal beliefs and practices that can be expressed with or without a specific formal religious belief.

The role of spirituality in treating chronic pain is vital as it helps patients to create a meaning and purpose that is essential in fighting chronic pain. Spirituality can help patients cope with the physical as well as the psychological component to chronic pain. The psychological meaning that patients assign to their pain impacts how they process their pain long term.

Spirituality lies in the sense of connection and inner strength and peace that individuals derive from the relationship with themselves, others, nature and possibly a connection to a specific religion. The role of a more spiritual patient is vital to improving a patient's overall well-being and quality of life. This improved well being takes time and training to accomplish but works through visualization, meditation, positive thinking and possibly even prayer.

A sense of connection to one's environment, nature and a higher power helps to give patient's an improved outlook on their treatment and significantly improved outcomes in treating their pain. Patients that find the ability to improve their inner strength will have an improved outlook, a sense of purpose and will lead them to a more effective treatment and success managing their chronic pain.

Food Intake

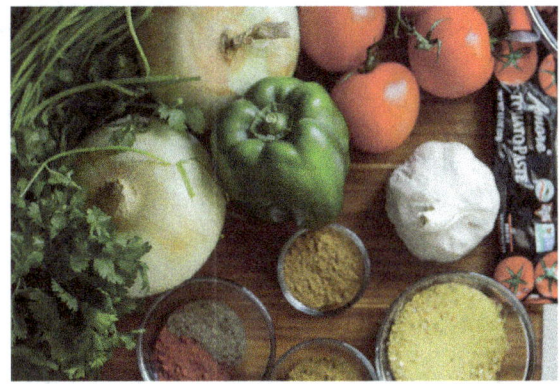

To make progress in finding an effective treatment for your fibromyalgia, every patient needs to evaluate the food they put into their body. Your food is the fuel your body uses to heal and to repair itself. There are countless studies that show direct correlation to increased inflammatory levels and increased pain with different food groups.

Here is a list of foods I recommend to avoid or consider a 6 week elimination trial.

#1 Avoid all sodas! Interesting enough, diet soft drinks, due to the sweetener Aspartame, seem to have even worse detrimental side effects for pain patients. I have seen dramatic results from patients eliminating all soft drinks and replacing with water. Eliminating soft drinks improves energy, decreases inflammatory levels that trigger or exacerbate Migraine Headaches, joint pain and Fibromyalgia.

#2 Limit or eliminate "Night shade" plants. Most patients assume that increasing vegetables would be a good lifestyle choice, however increasing studies are revealing that pain patients do worse with exposure to nightshade plants. Nightshade plants include a list of vegetables including tomatoes, peppers, white potatoes, eggplant and more! These nightshade plants increase inflammatory levels in the body and increase pain.

#3 Limit Carbohydrates! Carbs, specifically yeast related products worsen pain and specifically for Fibromyalgia patients.

#4 Avoid Fast food, not even going to explain this further.

#5 Do your best to shop the outer ring of the grocery store. The outer ring of the grocery store will have more of the food that should be put into our body. The inner aisles contain all the processed foods. Obviously it's impossible to avoid all of the inner aisles, but if you start on the outer ring you will improve your nutritional value.

#6 Consider being evaluated for Gluten sensitivity or allergy.

This list will give you a good starting point to cleaning up your food intake and improving the food that fuels your body.

Easy on the Carbs

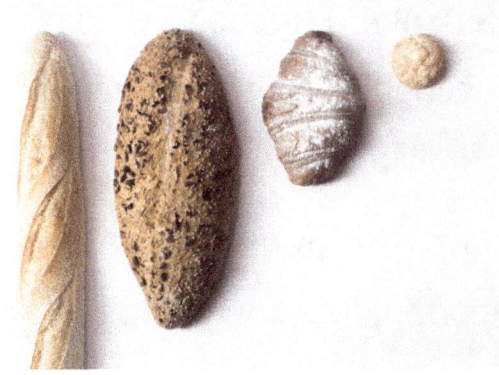

Carbohydrates make up the majority of the calories in many Americans' diets. Carbohydrates are a type of macro-nutrient which provide the body with energy. Grains such as bread, cereals, pasta and rices are all types of carbohydrates. Carbohydrates also come from fruits, vegetables and the natural sugars found in dairy products.

Some quick education on Carbs can help patients to have a better understanding of foods to be wary of in fighting chronic pain. Refined carbohydrates, such as white bread, white rice, cookies and candies, sodas, contain very little benefits to our general health. Refined carbs are low in fiber, vitamins and minerals. Complex carbohydrates such as whole wheat bread, brown rice, broccoli and asparagus, are rich in dietary fiber, help to stabilize blood sugar levels and are better choices for pain patients. Complex carbohydrates also contain high levels of vitamins and minerals.

Interesting enough most chronic pain patients, specifically Fibromyalgia patients, tend to have more frequent cravings for carbohydrates than healthy individuals. When patients give into the simple carbs they can enter a hypoglycemic state, or a sudden drop in blood sugar, perpetuating the fatigue and pain of Fibromyalgia and other chronic pain conditions.

Cutting out all carbohydrates from the diet is not recommended, since they do serve an important function in the metabolic process. Instead, I recommend cutting out all refined carbohydrates and choosing complex carbohydrates to make up 30% of your daily calorie intake.

These changes can significantly decrease inflammatory levels, improve energy and decrease pain.

Avoid Fast Food

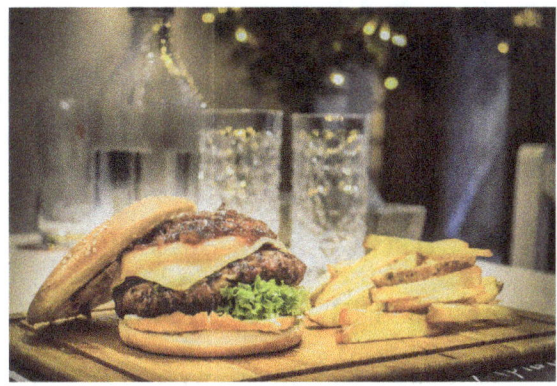

This is likely the most obvious of our recommendations for treating a patient's pain but also one of the most unlikely to be followed. Maybe it's our hectic lifestyle or just the fact that fast food is so cheap and convenient. Either way, patients inherently know that fast food is horrible for their general health and for pain but they just can't avoid it.

Fast food is not only quick to be prepared, but also contain some special group of fats that are known to be extremely harmful for the whole body, including for your joints. These fats, either saturated or trans can make the joints weaker and increase inflammatory markers. Alongside with trans and saturated fats, fast food contain high levels of sugar which also increases inflammatory markers and increases pain. Fast food also contains high levels of sodium, it is the main component of all non-organic pieces in a burger and usually it is the common ingredient that brings the whole taste to your meal.

Fast food with it's high levels of sodium, sugars, trans fats and carbohydrates combines to form what we like to call the pain bomb cocktail. This cocktail is further enhanced in Fibromyalgia patients as almost half Fibro patients suffer from Irritable Bowel Syndrome and leaky gut. Fast food also directly increases the likelihood of obesity and a sedentary lifestyle which in the long run will put more stress on joints and increase pain. Fast food will also increase the likeliness of heart disease and Type 2 Diabetes. Diabetic patients are at increased risk of peripheral neuropathies and chronic pain conditions.

Research an anti-inflammatory diet lifestyle and you will feel significantly better within a few weeks.

Avoid Nicotine

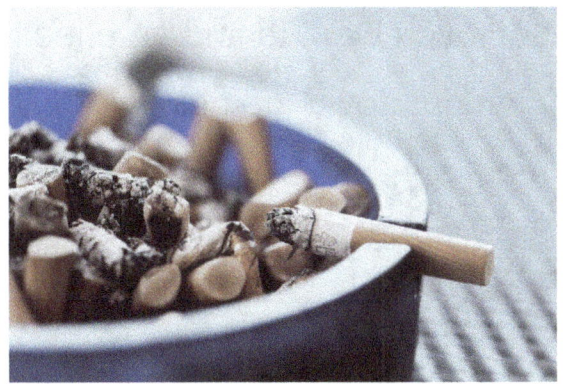

Over the past several years, increasing numbers of medical studies have shown the detrimental and negative effects of cigarette use and nicotine dependence on multiple aspects of health regarding the treatment of pain. Studies have shown that cigarette smoking and all other forms of nicotine consumption worsens the results of virtually all chronic pain treatments including cortisone injections and surgery. Also, everyone is well aware of the multitude of other health risks and expenses associated with nicotine consumption.

More recently, studies have shown an association between nicotine and the promotion of inflammation levels which directly worsen pain conditions and slow healing. Nicotine is a vasoconstrictor, shrinking blood vessels, which impacts oxygen perfusion to tissues and slows the body's own healing mechanisms and directly worsens pain and can led to further injury. Current research also reveals that nicotine acts as an accelerant to nerve related pain, similar to throwing gasoline on a fire.

Obviously, not all patients with fibromyalgia use nicotine products, but a good percentage do! If you want to find an effective treatment for your pain, you must first put down the nicotine so that you're not impeding your own recovery!

Anxiety and Depression

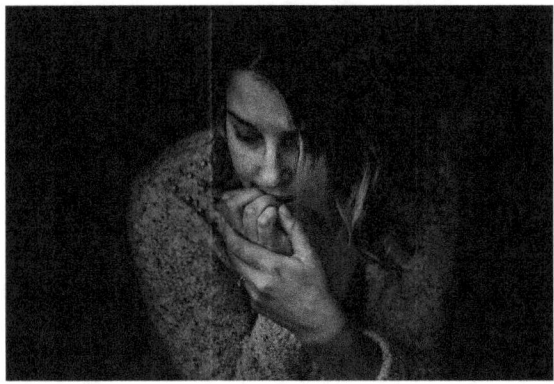

Chronic pain and depression are so closely linked that a viscous cycle can easily set in if one does not honestly address and treat any underlying depression. Studies show that patients with chronic pain have lower levels of the hormones serotonin and norepinephrine compared to patients not in pain. Lower levels of these hormones are known to lead to depression and anxiety. Combine these physiological lower levels of hormones with the frustration patient's feel regarding their lower quality of life and limitations from their pain and you have a set up for patients to fall into a feeling of hopelessness.

An important step towards finding an effective treatment for your pain is to work to attack depression directly. Depression is a medical condition that should be treated with a multi-modality approach. I work with our patients on setting up successful coping skills and techniques to improve their outlook on pain and depression. For a good amount of patients, working with a clinical psychologist or psychiatrist will also be a valuable member of a patient's pain fighting team. There are prescription medications that not only treat depression related issues but also have FDA indications for pain. Cymbalta is one example as it has FDA indications for Fibromyalgia, Diabetic peripheral neuropathy, chronic low back pain as well as anxiety and depression.

For patients that want to avoid traditional pharmacological medications, supplements like Magnesium have been used to treat stress and are an excellent smooth muscle relaxant. If you want to avoid pills all together, meditation and exercise are two successful strategies that every patient would benefit from. Both meditation and exercise boost endorphin levels, decrease stress hormone levels and give patients an improved outlook on life.

Finally, anyone with depression issues need to find someone to talk with, whether that be a support group, licensed professional, or a close friend. Releasing stress through the power of conversation is vital in helping patients gain both insight and learn tools to better cope with pain and depression.

Fibromyalgia 101

Let's put to the side the past stigmas associated with Fibromyalgia. For many years a majority of physicians did not believe in Fibromyalgia and there are still a few physicians who refuse to recognize or treat Fibro patients. While rounding on patients in the hospital, I have overhead a colleague label Fibromyalgia as the "depressed, overweight, middle age, housewife syndrome".

Luckily, the medical community is finally coming around to recognizing this chronic pain condition. Current Fibromyalgia research and treatment philosophy resolves around the theory of Fibromyalgia being a mixed component of a central nervous system dysfunction with a chronic myofascial component.

Fibromyalgia is a diagnosis of exclusion. It is important to make sure to have labs to rule our other connective tissues diseases first, like Rheumatoid Arthritis, before accepting the Fibro diagnosis.

Below is a list of recommendations I make to all of our Fibromyalgia patients on their first visit. After this list, I will then do a deep dive to explain each of these topics further:

1. Every Fibro patient needs a sleep study to treat any underlying sleep disorders that will directly complicate pain.

2. Treat any underlying depression, this can not be understated! Whether with counseling, psychiatric treatment, meditation and if needed medication

3. Check underlying vitamin deficiencies that can complicate pain, including Vitamin D, Vitamin B12, Vitamin B1, Vitamin B2 and Vitamin B6.

4. Start a daily home exercise/stretching program, Fibro will worsens with inactivity. I have heard every argument from patients that it hurts to much to exercise but it is critical to do some daily stretching/exercise routine. I recommend low impact yoga, pilates, tai chi, aquatic therapy.

5. Eliminate all soda's immediately, totally toxic and can increase inflammatory levels in the body complicating pain.

6. Restrict the 'nightshade plants' from the diet to limit their inflammatory related issues.

7. Limit yeast foods, so many of our patients struggle with this one but it will dramatically improve your energy

8. Work with a local physician and consider one of the FDA approved medications for Fibromyalgia: Cymbalta, Lyrica and Savella.

9. Consider low dose naltrexone trial. LDN is a game changer! Naltrexone works at the glial cells in the nervous system to help decrease nerve sensitivity.

Sleep Study

Sleep disturbances are a common and significant feature of fibromyalgia. Many individuals with fibromyalgia experience poor sleep quality, insomnia, and non-restorative sleep, which can exacerbate pain, fatigue, and other symptoms. Given the strong association between fibromyalgia and sleep disturbances, conducting a sleep study can provide valuable insights into the specific sleep-related issues that patients with fibromyalgia may be experiencing. This section explores the value of a sleep study in the evaluation and management of fibromyalgia patients.

A sleep study, also known as polysomnography, is a diagnostic test that monitors various physiological parameters during sleep. It is conducted in a specialized sleep laboratory or sometimes in the comfort of the patient's home using portable devices. By monitoring brain activity, eye movements, muscle tone, heart rate, and respiratory patterns, a sleep study can identify the presence of sleep disorders that may be contributing to the sleep disturbances in fibromyalgia patients.

Common sleep disorders that frequently coexist with fibromyalgia include obstructive sleep apnea, restless leg syndrome (RLS), periodic limb movement disorder (PLMD), and sleep-related bruxism (teeth grinding). Detecting and diagnosing these sleep disorders through a sleep study allows healthcare providers to implement targeted interventions to improve sleep quality and alleviate fibromyalgia symptoms.

A sleep study provides detailed information about the structure and quality of sleep. Sleep architecture refers to the different stages of sleep, including rapid eye movement (REM) sleep and non-rapid eye movement (NREM) sleep. By analyzing the sleep architecture, healthcare providers can identify abnormalities in the distribution and duration of sleep stages, as well as the presence of fragmented sleep.

In fibromyalgia patients, sleep studies often reveal disruptions in sleep architecture, such as decreased REM sleep, increased wakefulness during the night, and frequent arousals from deep sleep stages. These findings contribute to the understanding of the underlying mechanisms of fibromyalgia and help guide treatment strategies.

The information obtained from a sleep study can be instrumental in guiding treatment approaches for fibromyalgia patients. By identifying specific sleep disorders or abnormalities in sleep architecture, healthcare providers can tailor interventions to address these specific issues.

For instance, if obstructive sleep apnea is detected, continuous positive airway pressure (CPAP) therapy may be recommended to improve airflow and prevent airway obstructions during sleep. If restless leg syndrome or periodic limb movement disorder is diagnosed, medications or lifestyle modifications can be employed to alleviate these symptoms. Treatment options for sleep-related bruxism may involve dental devices or stress management techniques.

Moreover, improving sleep quality through targeted interventions can have a positive impact on overall fibromyalgia symptom management. Restorative sleep has been shown to reduce pain sensitivity, alleviate fatigue, and improve cognitive function in fibromyalgia patients.

In conclusion, a sleep study holds significant value in the evaluation and management of fibromyalgia patients. By identifying sleep disorders, assessing sleep architecture and quality, and guiding treatment approaches, sleep studies provide valuable insights into the specific sleep-related issues experienced by individuals with fibromyalgia. Addressing sleep disturbances can have a positive impact on overall fibromyalgia symptom management and improve the quality of life for these patients. Therefore, a sleep study should be considered as an important diagnostic tool for individuals with fibromyalgia to ensure comprehensive care and tailored treatment approaches.

Attack your Anxiety and Depression

Anxiety and depression are commonly reported comorbidities in individuals with fibromyalgia. The connection between fibromyalgia and these mental health conditions is complex and bidirectional, with each influencing the other. This section explores the relationship between fibromyalgia, anxiety, and depression and highlights the importance of addressing these mental health aspects in the management of fibromyalgia.

Anxiety and depression are prevalent in individuals with fibromyalgia, with research suggesting that up to 75% of fibromyalgia patients experience symptoms of anxiety or depression at some point. The exact nature of the relationship between fibromyalgia and these mental health conditions is still under investigation, but several factors contribute to their interplay.

On one hand, the chronic pain, fatigue, and other physical symptoms associated with fibromyalgia can lead to distress, frustration, and a reduced quality of life. Living with these symptoms day in and day out can contribute to the development or exacerbation of anxiety and depression. Moreover, the limitations and challenges imposed by fibromyalgia can lead to social isolation, loss of employment, and disrupted daily activities, further increasing the risk of developing anxiety and depression.

On the other hand, anxiety and depression can influence the

experience and perception of pain. These mental health conditions can amplify pain sensitivity, decrease pain tolerance, and contribute to the persistence of chronic pain. Anxiety can lead to hypervigilance towards bodily sensations, while depression can dampen mood and exacerbate feelings of helplessness and hopelessness, making pain management more challenging.

Addressing anxiety and depression in individuals with fibromyalgia is crucial for several reasons:

a) Improved Quality of Life: Anxiety and depression can significantly impair an individual's overall well-being and quality of life. By addressing these mental health conditions, individuals with fibromyalgia can experience a greater sense of emotional well-being, improved social functioning, and enhanced daily functioning.

b) Enhanced Pain Management: Anxiety and depression can exacerbate pain perception and make pain management less effective. Treating these mental health conditions can help reduce pain sensitivity, enhance the efficacy of pain management strategies, and improve overall pain control.

c) Breaking the Cycle: Anxiety, depression, and fibromyalgia can create a vicious cycle where one condition worsens the other. Treating anxiety and depression can help break this cycle, leading to a positive ripple effect on fibromyalgia symptoms and overall functioning.

The treatment of anxiety and depression in individuals with fibromyalgia typically involves a multidisciplinary approach. Some common treatment strategies include:

a) Psychotherapy: Cognitive-behavioral therapy (CBT) and other forms of psychotherapy have shown effectiveness in managing anxiety and depression in fibromyalgia patients. These therapies help individuals develop coping mechanisms, challenge negative thought patterns, and improve their overall psychological well-being.

b) Medications: Selective serotonin reuptake inhibitors (SSRIs), serotonin-norepinephrine reuptake inhibitors (SNRIs), and other antidepressant medications may be prescribed to alleviate symptoms of anxiety and depression. These medications can help regulate mood, reduce anxiety, and improve sleep quality.

c) Lifestyle Modifications: Incorporating healthy lifestyle practices such as regular exercise, stress management techniques (e.g., mindfulness, relaxation exercises), and improving sleep hygiene can have a positive impact on both mental health and fibromyalgia symptoms.

In conclusion, addressing anxiety and depression in individuals with fibromyalgia is essential for comprehensive and effective management of the condition. The bidirectional relationship between fibromyalgia and these mental health conditions necessitates a holistic approach.

Vitamin Deficiencies

There is a specific set of vitamin levels that I like to check in all patients who suffer from fibromyalgia. Too often these are overlooked and although on their own they are not the only cause of some patient's fibromyalgia pain, they definitely can complicate fibromyalgia pain.

Vitamin D is crucial for bone health, immune function, and overall well-being. Research suggests that individuals with fibromyalgia may have a higher prevalence of vitamin D deficiency compared to the general population. Vitamin D deficiency has been associated with increased pain sensitivity, muscle weakness, and fatigue, which are common symptoms in fibromyalgia.

Low levels of vitamin D have also been linked to an increased risk of developing chronic pain conditions, including fibromyalgia. Moreover, vitamin D deficiency can affect mood and cognitive function, contributing to the psychological symptoms experienced by individuals with fibromyalgia.

Vitamin B12 plays a vital role in neurological function, energy production, and red blood cell formation. Deficiency in vitamin B12 can lead to a range of symptoms, including fatigue, muscle weakness, cognitive impairment, and mood disturbances. These symptoms overlap with those experienced by individuals with fibromyalgia.

Some studies have found a higher prevalence of vitamin B12 deficiency in fibromyalgia patients compared to healthy individuals. While the exact relationship between vitamin B12 deficiency and fibromyalgia is not fully understood, addressing vitamin B12 deficiency through supplementation or dietary changes may help alleviate symptoms and improve overall well-being.

Magnesium is an essential mineral involved in numerous biochemical processes in the body, including muscle and nerve function, energy production, and regulation of mood. Low magnesium levels have been associated with increased pain sensitivity, muscle cramps, fatigue, and sleep disturbances.

Fibromyalgia patients often exhibit low magnesium levels, and magnesium supplementation has shown promise in reducing pain severity and improving sleep quality in some individuals with fibromyalgia. However, more research is needed to better understand the relationship between magnesium deficiency and fibromyalgia and to determine the optimal dosage and duration of magnesium supplementation.

In addition to vitamin D, B12, and magnesium, other vitamin deficiencies, such as vitamin B6 and vitamin E, have been suggested to contribute to fibromyalgia symptoms. Vitamin B6 deficiency can affect neurotransmitter function, potentially contributing to pain perception and mood disturbances. Vitamin E, as an antioxidant, may have a protective effect against oxidative stress and inflammation, which are implicated in fibromyalgia pathophysiology.

In conclusion, vitamin deficiencies, including vitamin D, B12, and magnesium, have been implicated in fibromyalgia and may contribute to the development and symptomatology of the condition. Addressing these deficiencies through supplementation or dietary modifications may help alleviate symptoms and improve the overall well-being of individuals with fibromyalgia.

The Value of Exercise

Exercise is recognized as a crucial component in the management of fibromyalgia. Regular physical activity has been shown to improve symptoms such as pain, fatigue, sleep disturbances, and overall quality of life in individuals with fibromyalgia. This section highlights the importance of a daily home exercise program for patients with fibromyalgia, emphasizing its benefits and considerations for implementation.

Engaging in a regular exercise program can help alleviate the symptoms associated with fibromyalgia. Exercise has been shown to reduce pain sensitivity, increase pain tolerance, and improve overall pain control in individuals with fibromyalgia. It helps to release endorphins, natural pain-relieving chemicals in the brain, which can enhance mood and promote a sense of well-being.

Regular physical activity can also combat fatigue, which is a common complaint in fibromyalgia. While it may seem counterintuitive, exercise has been found to boost energy levels and improve stamina in individuals with fibromyalgia. By gradually increasing activity levels, individuals can build strength, endurance, and resilience over time.

A daily home exercise program can improve physical functioning and enhance overall functional capacity in individuals with fibromyalgia. Regular exercise helps to increase muscle strength, flexibility, and cardiovascular fitness, which can lead to improved mobility, balance, and coordination. Enhanced physical functioning allows individuals to perform daily activities with greater ease and less discomfort.

Exercise also helps to prevent deconditioning and muscle atrophy, which can occur due to inactivity and sedentary behavior. By maintaining an active lifestyle, individuals can preserve muscle mass, joint flexibility, and overall physical health.

In addition to the physical benefits, a daily home exercise program can have significant psychological benefits for individuals with fibromyalgia. Exercise has been shown to improve mood, reduce symptoms of anxiety and depression, and enhance cognitive function in fibromyalgia patients.

Engaging in regular physical activity releases endorphins, which are natural mood-boosting chemicals. This can help alleviate symptoms of anxiety and depression commonly experienced by individuals with fibromyalgia. Exercise also promotes relaxation, stress reduction, and better sleep quality, all of which contribute to an improved psychological well-being.

When designing a home exercise program for individuals with fibromyalgia, it is important to consider certain factors:

a) Individualized Approach: Each person with fibromyalgia may have different abilities, limitations, and preferences. It is essential to tailor the exercise program to the individual's needs and abilities. Working with a healthcare professional or a qualified exercise specialist, such as a physical therapist, can help ensure a safe and effective exercise program.

b) Gradual Progression: Starting with low-impact, gentle exercises and gradually increasing intensity and duration is crucial to avoid exacerbating symptoms and causing undue stress on the body. Slow and steady progress allows individuals to build strength and endurance without overwhelming their system.

c) Variety and Flexibility: Incorporating a variety of exercises, including aerobic activities, strength training, and flexibility exercises, can provide a comprehensive workout and target different aspects of physical fitness. Additionally, allowing for flexibility in the exercise program, both in terms of scheduling and adapting exercises to accommodate fluctuations in symptoms, is important for long-term adherence.

In conclusion, a daily home exercise program is of utmost importance for individuals with fibromyalgia. Regular physical activity can significantly improve symptom management, enhance physical functioning, and provide psychological benefits. It is crucial to tailor the exercise program to individual needs, progress gradually, and incorporate variety and flexibility. By incorporating regular exercise into their daily routine, individuals with fibromyalgia can experience improved quality of life and better overall health and well-being.

Avoid Soda!

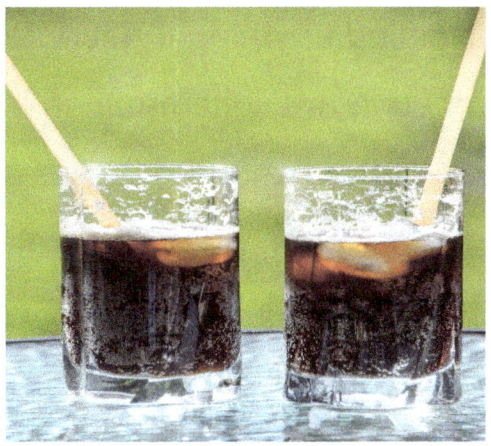

As discussed above, every patient with fibromyalgia will find tremendous improvement in eliminating soda.

There are specific 'drugs' in soda that activate the brain in these popular drinks like caffeine, sugar and flavor enhancers. More and more popular drinks are heavily loaded with caffeine, known to give people an energy boost and, when consumed regularly, these drinks also cause caffeine dependency.

The constant ups and downs of a caffeine roller coaster ride cause headaches, insomnia, mood instability and pain. Caffeine is a brain stimulant, a drug that can over-stimulate the brain and sometimes even cause death.

Sugar in soda is also a drug. Sugar not only stimulates the brain and causes dependency, it also harms the body in other ways. Complications from sugar include diabetes, a disease hallmarked by the harmful effects of frequent blood sugar spikes and consistently high blood sugar levels. Anyone who is experiencing pain should be extra cautious about avoiding anything that contains sugar because sugar promotes inflammation and inflammation leads to pain. In addition to sugar, sodas contain another, lesser known chemical that can lead to more pain, Aspartame. For years, researchers have reported about the potential harmful effects of Aspartame, a flavor enhancer. The effects are primarily seen in the nervous system such as: headaches, depression, anxiety and blurred vision. This chemical is meant to stimulate the taste buds but it appears to do more than that in some people. Aspartame could even contribute to a painful experience by sensitizing the nervous system.

Over the past 23 years, I have seen dramatic pain relief in patients who eliminate soda, specifically in patients who suffer from neuropathic pain and Fibromyalgia.

The Nightshade Plants

Nightshade plants belong to the Solanaceae family and include commonly consumed vegetables such as tomatoes, potatoes, peppers, and eggplants. In some alternative medicine circles, a theory has emerged suggesting that nightshade plants may exacerbate pain and inflammation in individuals with fibromyalgia. This section explores the relationship between nightshade plants and fibromyalgia pain, examining the available evidence and providing a balanced perspective on the topic.

One reason nightshade plants have been implicated in fibromyalgia pain is due to their content of alkaloids, particularly solanine and capsaicin. Alkaloids are natural compounds that can affect the nervous system and may have the potential to trigger or worsen pain and inflammation in some individuals.

Solanine, found in tomatoes, potatoes, and eggplants, is believed to have pro-inflammatory properties. Capsaicin, found in chili peppers, can cause a burning sensation and may activate pain receptors. It has been suggested that these alkaloids could contribute to increased pain sensitivity and symptoms in individuals with fibromyalgia.

It is essential to recognize that individuals with fibromyalgia may have different sensitivities and trigger foods. While some individuals may experience symptom exacerbation after consuming nightshade plants, others may not notice any adverse effects. Fibromyalgia is a complex condition with various contributing factors, and pain triggers can vary significantly among individuals.

Moreover, it is crucial to consider the overall dietary pattern and lifestyle factors in managing fibromyalgia. A balanced and varied diet, rich in fruits, vegetables, whole grains, lean proteins, and healthy fats, is generally recommended for optimal health. If an individual suspects that nightshade plants may worsen their symptoms, they can consider keeping a food diary and tracking their symptoms to identify potential triggers.

Is yeast a trigger?

In recent years, there has been growing interest in the potential effects of yeast on fibromyalgia pain. Some individuals with fibromyalgia report experiencing symptom exacerbation after consuming foods containing yeast or undergoing yeast-related treatments.

One hypothesis proposes that yeast overgrowth, particularly Candida albicans, may contribute to fibromyalgia symptoms. Candida albicans is a type of yeast that naturally resides in the human body, typically in the gut, without causing harm. However, under certain conditions, such as a weakened immune system or imbalanced gut microbiota, Candida overgrowth can occur, leading to a condition called systemic candidiasis.

Systemic candidiasis is characterized by an overgrowth of Candida throughout the body, including the digestive tract. It has been suggested that the byproducts of Candida metabolism, such as acetaldehyde, may trigger inflammation and worsen fibromyalgia symptoms, including pain, fatigue, and cognitive difficulties.

It is essential to consider other factors that may contribute to symptom exacerbation in individuals who suspect yeast-related issues. Fibromyalgia is a complex condition influenced by various factors, including stress, sleep disturbances, dietary patterns, and individual sensitivities. It is possible that some individuals with fibromyalgia may have sensitivities or allergies to yeast-containing foods, which can contribute to symptom exacerbation. In such cases, avoiding or reducing the consumption of yeast-containing foods may provide relief.

The 3 FDA Approved Medications

Fibromyalgia is a chronic condition characterized by widespread pain, fatigue, sleep disturbances, and cognitive difficulties. Managing fibromyalgia can be challenging, and medications are often prescribed to help alleviate symptoms and improve quality of life. Cymbalta, Savella, and Lyrica are three medications commonly used in the treatment of fibromyalgia. This section explores the benefits of these medications and how they work differently in managing fibromyalgia symptoms.

1. Cymbalta (Duloxetine):

Cymbalta, also known by its generic name duloxetine, is an antidepressant that belongs to a class of medications called serotonin-norepinephrine reuptake inhibitors (SNRIs). It works by increasing the levels of serotonin and norepinephrine, two neurotransmitters involved in mood regulation and pain perception.

Benefits of Cymbalta for Fibromyalgia:

- Pain Relief: Cymbalta has been shown to reduce pain severity in individuals with fibromyalgia. It helps modulate pain signals in the central nervous system, making individuals more tolerant to pain.
- Improved Mood: Cymbalta can help alleviate symptoms of depression and anxiety, which commonly coexist with

fibromyalgia. By balancing serotonin levels, it may improve mood and overall well-being.

- Enhanced Sleep Quality: Cymbalta can help regulate sleep patterns and improve sleep quality in individuals with fibromyalgia, which is crucial for managing fatigue and promoting restorative sleep.

2. Savella (Milnacipran):

Savella, or milnacipran, is another medication that belongs to the SNRI class. Similar to Cymbalta, it works by increasing the levels of serotonin and norepinephrine in the brain. It is specifically approved for the treatment of fibromyalgia.

Benefits of Savella for Fibromyalgia:

- Pain Reduction: Savella has been shown to reduce pain intensity and improve overall pain control in individuals with fibromyalgia. It helps normalize pain processing in the central nervous system.
- Increased Physical Functioning: Savella can improve physical functioning, including walking ability and overall functional capacity, in individuals with fibromyalgia. This can enhance mobility and improve daily functioning.
- Reduced Fatigue: Savella may help alleviate fatigue, one of the most debilitating symptoms of fibromyalgia. By modulating

neurotransmitters involved in energy regulation, it can boost energy levels and combat fibromyalgia-related fatigue.

3. Lyrica (Pregabalin):

Lyrica, or pregabalin, is an anticonvulsant medication that also acts as a neuropathic pain agent. It works by binding to certain calcium channels in the central nervous system, reducing the release of neurotransmitters involved in pain signaling.

Benefits of Lyrica for Fibromyalgia:

- Pain Relief: Lyrica has been shown to effectively reduce pain severity and improve pain control in individuals with fibromyalgia. It can help decrease pain sensitivity and improve overall pain management.
- Improved Sleep: Lyrica can improve sleep quality and reduce sleep disturbances in individuals with fibromyalgia. By promoting better sleep, it can contribute to overall symptom improvement.
- Anxiety Reduction: Lyrica may help alleviate symptoms of anxiety that often accompany fibromyalgia. By modulating neurotransmitter activity, it can have a calming effect and improve overall mood.

Differences in Mechanism of Action:

Although Cymbalta, Savella, and Lyrica all aim to manage fibromyalgia symptoms, they work differently in the body:

- Cymbalta and Savella primarily increase the levels of serotonin and norepinephrine,
- Lyrica, on the other hand, works by binding to calcium channels and reducing the release of certain neurotransmitters involved in pain signaling.

Low Dose Naltrexone (LDN)

Fibromyalgia is a complex chronic condition characterized by widespread pain, fatigue, sleep disturbances, and cognitive difficulties. While the exact cause of fibromyalgia is still not fully understood, emerging research suggests that dysregulation of the immune system and abnormal pain processing in the central nervous system play a role. Low dose naltrexone (LDN) is a medication that has gained attention in recent years for its potential benefits in managing fibromyalgia symptoms. This section explores the benefits of LDN, describes dosing considerations, and explains how LDN targets glial cells and their relation to nerve pain in fibromyalgia.

1. Benefits of Low Dose Naltrexone for Fibromyalgia:

LDN is an opioid receptor antagonist that, at low doses, has been found to have immunomodulatory and analgesic effects. While more research is needed to fully understand its mechanisms of action, several potential benefits of LDN for fibromyalgia have been reported:

- Pain Reduction: LDN has shown promise in reducing pain severity in individuals with fibromyalgia. It may help modulate pain signaling pathways and decrease pain sensitivity.
- Improved Sleep Quality: Many individuals with fibromyalgia struggle with sleep disturbances. LDN has been reported to improve sleep quality and promote more restorative sleep.

- Enhanced Mood and Well-being: LDN has been associated with improvements in mood, including reductions in depression and anxiety symptoms. It may contribute to an overall sense of well-being and improved quality of life.

2. Dosing Considerations for Low Dose Naltrexone:

The term "low dose" refers to the use of naltrexone at significantly lower doses than those typically used for opioid addiction or alcohol dependence. While standard doses of naltrexone range from 50 to 100 mg, low doses for conditions like fibromyalgia usually range from 1.5 to 4.5 mg.

LDN is typically taken orally once daily at bedtime. Starting with a low dose, usually around 1.5 mg, allows the body to gradually adjust to the medication and minimize potential side effects. If necessary, the dosage can be gradually increased over time, under the guidance of a healthcare professional, to achieve the optimal therapeutic effect.

3. Targeting Glial Cells and their Relation to Nerve Pain:

Glial cells, also known as neuroglia, are non-neuronal cells that provide support and protection to neurons in the central nervous system. They play a crucial role in maintaining the normal functioning of the nervous system. In the context of fibromyalgia, glial cells have been implicated in the amplification of pain signals and the development of chronic pain. The glial cells have been called the glue of the nervous system.

Research suggests that glial cells, specifically microglia and astrocytes, become activated and release pro-inflammatory substances in response to injury or chronic pain conditions. This activation contributes to a state of neuroinflammation, leading to increased pain sensitivity and perpetuation of the pain cycle.

Low dose naltrexone is thought to modulate glial cell activity by blocking opioid receptors on these cells. This blockade can lead to a decrease in pro-inflammatory substances released by glial cells, helping to reduce neuroinflammation and alleviate pain.

Low dose naltrexone (LDN) has been an absolute game changer for my patients. It should be noted that Low dose naltrexone should not be combined with traditional opioid medications. I also like to discuss with my Fibro patients that you need to give LDN time to work, I classically like patients to commit to a 6 week trial before passing judgement on the medication.

Muscle Relaxers

Managing the symptoms of fibromyalgia can be challenging, and healthcare providers often employ various approaches to help alleviate pain and improve quality of life. One such approach involves the use of muscle relaxers. In this section, we will explore the potential benefits of muscle relaxers for individuals with fibromyalgia.

Muscle relaxers, also known as skeletal muscle relaxants, are medications that work by reducing muscle spasms and tension. In fibromyalgia, individuals often experience persistent muscle pain, stiffness, and spasms, which can significantly impact their daily functioning. Muscle relaxers can provide relief by relaxing the muscles and relieving the associated pain.

By targeting the muscle fibers and decreasing muscle tension, these medications can help alleviate the muscular component of fibromyalgia pain. This can lead to improved mobility, increased physical activity, and an overall reduction in discomfort. Muscle stiffness is a common complaint among individuals with fibromyalgia. It can make movement challenging and contribute to the overall pain experienced. Muscle relaxers can help decrease muscle stiffness by promoting muscle relaxation and improving flexibility.

By inhibiting the signals that cause muscle contractions and reducing muscle tone, muscle relaxers allow for greater ease of movement and can help individuals with fibromyalgia regain some range of motion.

This, in turn, may contribute to improved functioning and a better overall quality of life.

Sleep disturbances are prevalent among individuals with fibromyalgia, and muscle pain and tension can exacerbate sleep difficulties. Muscle relaxers can help address this issue by promoting relaxation and easing muscle-related discomfort, thereby improving sleep quality.

By reducing muscle spasms and tension, muscle relaxers can contribute to a more restful sleep experience. This is particularly important for individuals with fibromyalgia, as quality sleep plays a vital role in managing fatigue, restoring energy levels, and supporting overall well-being.

Muscle relaxers can also complement other treatments commonly used for fibromyalgia. For example, when used in conjunction with physical therapy, muscle relaxers can help facilitate the therapeutic process by reducing muscle tension and allowing for greater flexibility during exercises and stretches. This can enhance the effectiveness of physical therapy interventions and improve functional outcomes.

Furthermore, muscle relaxers may also enhance the response to other pain management strategies, such as analgesic medications or non-pharmacological interventions. By targeting the muscular component of fibromyalgia pain, muscle relaxers can work synergistically with other treatments to provide comprehensive relief.

In conclusion, muscle relaxers offer potential benefits for individuals with fibromyalgia by alleviating muscle pain, reducing stiffness, improving sleep quality, and enhancing the response to other treatments. These medications can help relax muscles, promote flexibility, and contribute to an overall reduction in discomfort and improved functionality.

TCA

Fibromyalgia is a complex chronic condition characterized by widespread pain, fatigue, sleep disturbances, and cognitive difficulties. Managing fibromyalgia symptoms often requires a multimodal approach, and one class of medications that has shown potential benefit is tricyclic antidepressants (TCAs). In this section, we will explore the potential benefits of TCAs for individuals with fibromyalgia and discuss some of the most commonly prescribed TCAs for this condition.

One of the primary reasons TCAs are prescribed for fibromyalgia is their potential to provide pain relief. TCAs work by increasing the levels of certain neurotransmitters, such as serotonin and norepinephrine, in the brain. These neurotransmitters play a role in modulating pain perception and can help reduce the intensity and sensitivity of pain signals.

By altering the balance of neurotransmitters, TCAs can help alleviate the widespread musculoskeletal pain associated with fibromyalgia. This pain relief can improve overall quality of life and enable individuals to engage in daily activities with less discomfort.

Sleep disturbances are common in fibromyalgia, with individuals often experiencing difficulties falling asleep, staying asleep, or achieving restorative sleep. TCAs have sedative properties that can help regulate sleep patterns and promote better sleep quality.

By enhancing sleep architecture and promoting deeper, more restful sleep, TCAs can address the sleep disturbances that contribute to the fatigue and cognitive difficulties experienced by individuals with fibromyalgia. Improved sleep can also positively impact pain perception and overall well-being.

Depression and anxiety commonly coexist with fibromyalgia, and TCAs can help address these comorbid mood disorders. TCAs have been used for decades to treat depression, and their effects on serotonin and norepinephrine can improve mood and emotional well-being.

By alleviating symptoms of depression and anxiety, TCAs can contribute to an overall improvement in the psychological and emotional aspects of fibromyalgia. This can lead to a more positive outlook, increased resilience, and a better ability to cope with the challenges of living with fibromyalgia.

While individual responses to TCAs may vary, some of the most commonly prescribed TCAs for fibromyalgia include:

- Amitriptyline: Amitriptyline is often the first choice among TCAs for fibromyalgia. It has demonstrated effectiveness in reducing pain, improving sleep quality, and alleviating other associated symptoms. It is usually started at a low dose and gradually titrated upward based on individual response and tolerability.

- Nortriptyline: Nortriptyline is a TCA closely related to amitriptyline. It is often used as an alternative to amitriptyline, especially in individuals who may experience intolerable side effects with amitriptyline. Nortriptyline is generally better tolerated and has similar pain-relieving and sleep-improving effects.

Opioid Medication

Fibromyalgia is a chronic condition characterized by widespread pain, fatigue, and other associated symptoms. Managing fibromyalgia pain can be challenging, and healthcare providers often explore various treatment options, including opioid medications. Opioids are powerful pain relievers that can provide significant relief for acute and chronic pain conditions. However, their use in fibromyalgia remains a topic of debate due to the potential risks and concerns associated with long-term opioid therapy. In this section, we will examine the pros and cons of using opioid medication for fibromyalgia pain management.

Pros of Using Opioid Medication:

1. Pain Relief: Opioids are potent analgesics and can effectively reduce pain severity in individuals with fibromyalgia. They work by binding to opioid receptors in the central nervous system, altering the perception of pain and providing relief. For some individuals, opioids may provide temporary respite from intense fibromyalgia pain, enhancing their overall quality of life.

2. Improved Functioning: By reducing pain, opioids may improve physical functioning and mobility for individuals with fibromyalgia. This can lead to increased activity levels, improved participation in daily activities, and enhanced overall well-being. Opioids may enable individuals to engage in exercises and physical therapies that were previously unattainable due to

severe pain.

3. Enhanced Sleep: Sleep disturbances are common in fibromyalgia, and opioids can help improve sleep quality by reducing pain and promoting relaxation. Restorative sleep is essential for managing fibromyalgia symptoms, as it aids in alleviating fatigue and cognitive difficulties associated with the condition.

Cons of Using Opioid Medication:

1. Risk of Addiction and Dependency: Opioids are highly addictive substances, and long-term use increases the risk of developing dependence or addiction. Fibromyalgia is a chronic condition that requires ongoing management, and the potential for dependence poses a significant concern. Individuals may develop tolerance to opioids, requiring higher doses to achieve the same pain relief, and discontinuing opioid therapy can result in withdrawal symptoms.

2. Side Effects and Adverse Reactions: Opioids can cause various side effects, including constipation, nausea, drowsiness, cognitive impairment, and respiratory depression. These side effects can significantly impact quality of life and overall functioning. Additionally, individuals with fibromyalgia may be more susceptible to experiencing adverse reactions to opioids

due to their heightened sensitivity to medications.

3. Long-Term Safety Concerns: Prolonged use of opioids is associated with numerous long-term safety concerns. These include the potential for opioid overdose, respiratory depression, hormonal imbalances, immune system suppression, and increased susceptibility to infections. Furthermore, the use of opioids in fibromyalgia has not been extensively studied, and the long-term effects of opioid therapy on fibromyalgia symptoms and disease progression are unclear.

4. Negative Impact on Mental Health: Opioids can exacerbate mood disorders such as depression and anxiety, which often coexist with fibromyalgia. Additionally, the psychological burden of relying on opioids for pain relief, the fear of addiction, and the stigma surrounding opioid use can contribute to increased stress, anxiety, and emotional distress.

5. Interference with Cognitive Function: Fibromyalgia is already associated with cognitive difficulties, commonly referred to as "fibro fog." Opioids can further impair cognitive function, leading to difficulties with memory, attention, and concentration. This can have a significant impact on daily activities, work productivity, and overall quality of life.

Associated medical conditions

Now that I have covered the history, current theory, general recommendations and lifestyle modifications for Fibromyalgia; it is now time to turn our focus towards commonly associated conditions and their treatment. Here is a list of the most common conditions associated with Fibromyalgia and then we will do a deep dive into each one of them with their own chapter.

Here are the top 10 conditions commonly associated with fibromyalgia patients:

1. Chronic Fatigue Syndrome (CFS): Fibromyalgia and chronic fatigue syndrome often coexist, and many individuals with fibromyalgia also experience persistent fatigue, weakness, and reduced stamina.

2. Irritable Bowel Syndrome (IBS): Fibromyalgia and IBS frequently occur together, leading to symptoms such as abdominal pain, bloating, diarrhea, and constipation. The combination of these conditions can significantly impact gastrointestinal function and quality of life.

3. Migraines and Headaches: Individuals with fibromyalgia often report frequent migraines or tension headaches. The exact relationship between fibromyalgia and headaches is not fully understood, but the coexistence of these conditions can

contribute to increased pain and discomfort.

4. Temporomandibular Joint (TMJ) Disorders: TMJ disorders involve dysfunction and pain in the jaw joint and surrounding muscles. Many individuals with fibromyalgia experience TMJ symptoms, including jaw pain, difficulty chewing, and jaw clicking or locking.

5. Depression and Anxiety: Fibromyalgia is often associated with mood disorders such as depression and anxiety. The chronic pain and fatigue experienced in fibromyalgia can significantly impact mental health, leading to emotional distress and reduced quality of life.

6. Sleep Disorders: Sleep disturbances are common in fibromyalgia, and conditions like insomnia and sleep apnea frequently coexist. These sleep disorders can further contribute to fatigue, cognitive difficulties, and overall impairment in fibromyalgia patients.

7. Rheumatoid Arthritis (RA): Fibromyalgia and rheumatoid arthritis share overlapping symptoms, and it is not uncommon for individuals with RA to also have fibromyalgia. The presence of both conditions can complicate pain management and treatment strategies.

8. Lupus: Systemic lupus erythematosus (SLE) and fibromyalgia

can present with similar symptoms, including fatigue, joint pain, and muscle pain. Distinguishing between the two conditions can be challenging, and some individuals may experience both simultaneously.

9. Osteoarthritis (OA): Fibromyalgia can occur alongside osteoarthritis, a degenerative joint disease characterized by joint pain and stiffness. The coexistence of fibromyalgia and OA can lead to increased pain and functional limitations.

10. Endometriosis: Fibromyalgia and endometriosis commonly occur together, particularly in women. Endometriosis involves the growth of uterine tissue outside the uterus, leading to chronic pelvic pain, painful menstruation, and other associated symptoms.

It's important to note that the presence of these conditions can vary among individuals with fibromyalgia, and not every individual will experience all of these associated conditions. Proper diagnosis, comprehensive medical evaluation, and individualized treatment plans are crucial for addressing the complex needs of individuals with fibromyalgia and its associated conditions.

Chronic Fatigue Syndrome

Chronic Fatigue Syndrome (CFS), also known as myalgic encephalomyelitis (ME), is a complex and debilitating condition characterized by persistent fatigue that is not alleviated by rest and is accompanied by a range of other symptoms. While the exact cause of CFS remains unclear, treatment approaches focus on symptom management and improving quality of life.

The treatment of CFS typically involves a multidisciplinary approach, addressing the various symptoms experienced by individuals. The primary goals are to alleviate symptoms, improve function, and enhance overall well-being. Some of the symptom-based treatment approaches include:

a. Cognitive Behavioral Therapy (CBT): CBT is a type of therapy that helps individuals change negative thought patterns and develop effective coping strategies. It has been shown to be beneficial in managing symptoms of CFS, including fatigue, pain, and sleep disturbances.

b. Graded Exercise Therapy (GET): GET involves gradually increasing physical activity levels under the guidance of a healthcare professional. It aims to improve fitness and tolerance to exercise without exacerbating symptoms. However, it is essential to individualize exercise programs based on an individual's capabilities and avoid overexertion.

c. Sleep Management: Addressing sleep disturbances is crucial in CFS management. Strategies may include establishing a consistent sleep schedule, improving sleep hygiene, and addressing any underlying sleep disorders, such as sleep apnea or insomnia.

Medications can be used to manage specific symptoms and provide relief in some cases of CFS. However, it's important to note that medication options for CFS are limited, and the response to medication can vary among individuals. Some medications that may be prescribed for symptom management in CFS include:

a. Pain Medications: Over-the-counter pain relievers (e.g., acetaminophen) or prescription medications (e.g., low-dose tricyclic antidepressants) may be used to alleviate pain associated with CFS.

b. Sleep Aids: In cases of severe sleep disturbances, sleep aids or medications that promote better sleep may be prescribed to improve sleep quality.

c. Symptom-Specific Medications: Depending on the symptoms experienced by an individual with CFS, medications such as anti-nausea drugs, antihistamines, or antidepressants may be prescribed to target specific symptoms.

Lifestyle modifications play a vital role in managing CFS symptoms and improving overall well-being. These may include:

a. Energy Conservation: Learning to manage energy levels and avoid overexertion is essential in CFS management. Pacing activities, taking regular breaks, and prioritizing tasks can help conserve energy and prevent symptom flare-ups.

b. Stress Management: Stress can exacerbate CFS symptoms, so stress management techniques, such as relaxation exercises, meditation, and mindfulness, may be helpful in reducing stress levels.

  c. Dietary Adjustments: Some individuals with CFS report improvements in symptoms by making dietary changes, such as avoiding certain food triggers or following specific dietary plans. However, more research is needed to establish the effectiveness of dietary interventions for CFS.

Migraines

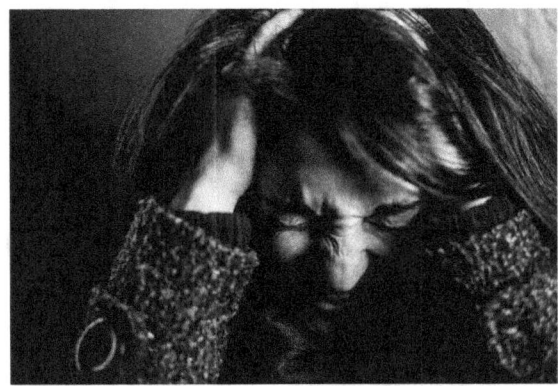

Migraine headaches are a common and debilitating condition that affects millions of people worldwide. Migraines are characterized by severe headaches, accompanied by a range of symptoms, including nausea, sensitivity to light and sound, and visual disturbances. The exact cause of migraines is not fully understood, but it is believed to be related to a combination of genetic and environmental factors. There are several treatment options available for migraine headaches, including pharmacological and non-pharmacological therapies. In the next few chapters, I will provide an overview of the current treatment options for migraine headaches.

Pharmacological treatments for migraines are the most commonly used and include over-the-counter pain relievers, such as acetaminophen, and prescription medications, such as triptans and nonsteroidal anti-inflammatory drugs (NSAIDs). Triptans are a type of medication specifically designed to treat migraines, and they work by narrowing the blood vessels in the brain and reducing inflammation. NSAIDs, such as ibuprofen, can also be used to relieve migraine pain.

Preventative medications are also used to reduce the frequency and severity of migraines. These medications include beta-blockers, calcium channel blockers, and anticonvulsants, CGRP Inhibitors among others. Preventative medications can help to reduce the number of migraines a person experiences, making it easier to manage the condition.

Non-pharmacological treatments for migraines include lifestyle changes, such as regular exercise, stress management techniques, and dietary changes. Keeping a migraine diary can also be helpful in identifying triggers, such as certain foods or environmental factors, that may contribute to migraines.

Cognitive-behavioral therapy (CBT) and biofeedback are two forms of therapy that have been shown to be effective in managing migraines. CBT helps individuals to identify and manage negative thought patterns and behaviors that may contribute to migraines, while biofeedback helps individuals to understand and control the physical responses associated with migraines.

Interventional techniques, such as nerve blocks, SPG and Botox injections, may also be used to manage migraines. Nerve blocks are used to block pain signals to the brain, while Botox injections can help to relax the muscles that are associated with migraines.

Finally, complementary and alternative therapies, such as acupuncture, massage, and herbal remedies, may also be used to manage migraines. These therapies can provide natural and non-invasive ways to relieve migraine pain and may be used in conjunction with other treatments.

In conclusion, there are several effective treatment options available for migraine headaches. A combination of pharmacological and non-pharmacological therapies, along with interventional techniques and complementary and alternative therapies, can provide effective relief for individuals suffering from migraines. It is important to work with a healthcare provider to determine the best approach for managing migraines and to ensure safe and effective pain relief.

CGRP

CGRP inhibitors are a novel new treatment for Headaches Calcitonin gene-related peptide (CGRP) is a neuropeptide that is involved in the regulation of pain, particularly in the management of headache disorders. Over the past few years, there has been a growing interest in the use of CGRP inhibitors as a treatment option for headaches, including migraines. This essay will provide a comprehensive overview of CGRP, its role in headaches, and the current status of CGRP-based treatments for headaches.

CGRP is a peptide hormone that is produced and released by sensory neurons in response to various triggers. It acts as a vasodilator, causing the blood vessels in the head to expand, leading to increased blood flow and inflammation. CGRP is also involved in the transmission of pain signals from the periphery to the central nervous system. It has been found to play a key role in the pathophysiology of migraines and other types of headaches.

There are two main types of CGRP inhibitors: monoclonal antibodies (mAbs) and small molecule drugs. mAbs work by binding to CGRP in the bloodstream, preventing it from reaching the blood vessels and reducing inflammation. Small molecule drugs, on the other hand, block the CGRP receptors, preventing CGRP from binding and activating the receptors.

CGRP inhibitors have shown promise in the treatment of migraines and other types of headaches. Clinical trials have shown that CGRP inhibitors are effective in reducing the frequency and severity of migraines, as well as reducing the use of rescue medications. The benefits of CGRP inhibitors have also been demonstrated in patients with cluster headaches, a rare but debilitating form of headache.

One of the most promising CGRP inhibitors is erenumab (Aimovig), which is a monoclonal antibody that has been approved by the US Food and Drug Administration (FDA) for the treatment of migraines. Erenumab is administered as a subcutaneous injection and has been shown to reduce the frequency and severity of migraines by 50% or more in some patients. Another CGRP inhibitor, fremanezumab (Ajovy), has also been approved by the FDA for the treatment of migraines. It is administered as a subcutaneous injection and has been shown to reduce the frequency of migraines by 50% or more in some patients.

Small molecule CGRP inhibitors are also being developed and tested for the treatment of headaches. One of the most promising of these drugs is ubrogepant (Ubrelvy), which has been approved by the FDA for the treatment of acute migraines. Ubrogepant is taken orally and has been shown to provide rapid and effective relief from migraine symptoms.

In addition to the benefits in the management of headaches, CGRP inhibitors have also been shown to have positive effects on other conditions, such as cardiovascular disease and stroke. CGRP has been found to play a role in the development of these conditions, and the inhibition of CGRP may help to prevent or manage them.

Botox for Migraine

Botulinum toxin type A, commonly known as Botox, is a popular and effective treatment option for individuals suffering from headaches. Botox works by temporarily blocking the release of chemicals that transmit pain signals in the brain. This reduces the frequency and severity of headaches, providing relief for individuals who suffer from chronic migraines, tension headaches, and other types of headaches. In this essay, we will provide an overview of the current uses of Botox for headache treatment and its potential benefits and risks.

Botox has been used as a treatment for headaches for over two decades, and its effectiveness has been widely documented in numerous clinical studies. The American Migraine Foundation and the American Academy of Neurology have both endorsed the use of Botox for the treatment of chronic migraines. Botox is typically administered through a series of injections into specific muscle groups, and the treatment usually takes less than 30 minutes. The effects of Botox can last for up to three months, and the treatment can be repeated as needed.

One of the primary benefits of Botox for headache treatment is its ability to reduce the frequency and severity of headaches. In clinical studies, individuals who received Botox injections for their headaches experienced a significant reduction in the number of headaches per month compared to those who received a placebo. Additionally, Botox has been shown to improve quality of life and reduce the use of other headache medications, such as pain relievers and triptans.

Another benefit of Botox for headache treatment is its low risk profile. Botox has been used for cosmetic purposes for over 20 years and has a well-established safety record. The most common side effects of Botox for headache treatment are mild, such as temporary muscle weakness or soreness at the injection site, and they typically resolve on their own within a few days. Serious side effects are rare, but as with any medical procedure, it is important to discuss potential risks with a healthcare provider before undergoing treatment.

It is important to note that Botox is not a cure for headaches, but rather a tool for managing symptoms. Individuals who receive Botox for their headaches may still experience occasional headaches, but the frequency and severity of these headaches are usually significantly reduced. Additionally, Botox does not work for everyone, and some individuals may not experience the full benefits of treatment.

In conclusion, Botox is a safe and effective treatment option for individuals suffering from headaches. Its ability to reduce the frequency and severity of headaches, improve quality of life, and low risk profile make it an attractive option for those seeking relief from chronic migraines, tension headaches, and other types of headaches.

As with any medical procedure, it is important to discuss the potential benefits and risks with a healthcare provider and to determine the best approach for managing headaches. With ongoing research and advancements in headache treatment, Botox will likely continue to play a significant role in the management of headaches for years to come.

SPG

The sphenopalatine ganglion (SPG) is a group of nerve cells located in the back of the nasal cavity that is believed to play a significant role in the development of certain types of headaches. The SPG has been targeted for treatment in recent years due to its potential for providing relief for headaches, including migraines and cluster headaches. In this essay, we will provide an overview of the current treatments for headaches using SPG stimulation.

One of the most common methods of SPG stimulation is a procedure called the Sphenopalatine Ganglion (SPG) Block. This is a minimally invasive procedure that involves the non needle catheter directed procedure of a local anesthetic into the nasal cavity to block the SPG and provide relief from headaches. This procedure is typically performed in an outpatient setting and can provide quick relief for headache pain.

In practice, I have seen SPG as a very successful treatment not only for headaches but various atypical facial pains, cluster headaches and even trigeminal neuralgia.

TMJ

The temporomandibular joint (TMJ) is the joint that connects the jawbone to the skull, allowing for movement necessary for chewing, speaking, and other oral functions. TMJ disorders can cause pain, discomfort, and dysfunction in the jaw joint and surrounding muscles. The treatment of TMJ disorders aims to alleviate symptoms, improve jaw function, and enhance overall quality of life.

In mild cases of TMJ disorders, self-care measures and lifestyle modifications may be sufficient to relieve symptoms. These can include:

a. Applying Heat or Cold Packs: Applying warm or cold compresses to the jaw joint can help alleviate pain and reduce inflammation.

b. Soft Diet: Eating soft, easy-to-chew foods can reduce stress on the jaw joint and muscles, giving them time to heal.

c. Jaw Exercises: Gentle jaw exercises and stretching techniques can help improve jaw mobility and strengthen the muscles surrounding the TMJ.

d. Stress Reduction: Stress can contribute to TMJ symptoms, so techniques such as relaxation exercises, stress management, and avoiding activities that cause excessive jaw clenching or teeth grinding can be beneficial.

Medications may be used in conjunction with self-care measures to manage pain and inflammation associated with TMJ disorders. Some common medications used in the treatment of TMJ disorders include:

a. Nonsteroidal Anti-Inflammatory Drugs (NSAIDs): Over-the-counter NSAIDs, such as ibuprofen or naproxen, can help reduce pain and inflammation in the TMJ area.

b. Muscle Relaxants: Prescription muscle relaxants may be prescribed to relieve muscle tension and spasms in the jaw.

c. Tricyclic Antidepressants: In some cases, tricyclic antidepressants can help alleviate pain associated with TMJ disorders. These medications work by altering the perception of pain signals.

Dental interventions are commonly used in the treatment of TMJ disorders. These may include:

a. Oral Splints or Mouthguards: Custom-fitted oral splints or mouthguards are often used to help stabilize the jaw and reduce pressure on the TMJ. They can be particularly helpful for individuals who clench or grind their teeth at night.

b. Dental Corrections: Dental treatments, such as orthodontic adjustments or dental restorations, may be recommended to correct misaligned teeth or improve the bite, which can contribute to TMJ disorders.

Physical therapy can play a significant role in the treatment of TMJ disorders. A physical therapist specializing in TMJ disorders may employ various techniques, including:

a. Jaw Exercises: Specific exercises to strengthen the jaw muscles and improve joint mobility.

b. Manual Therapy: Hands-on techniques, such as massage or mobilization, to relieve muscle tension and improve joint function.

c. Posture and Body Mechanics: Education on proper posture and body mechanics to reduce strain on the jaw joint and muscles.

In severe cases of TMJ disorders that do not respond to conservative treatments, invasive interventions may be considered. These interventions are typically reserved for individuals with significant pain and functional limitations. Examples include:

a. Injections: Corticosteroid injections into the TMJ can provide temporary relief from pain and inflammation.

b. Arthrocentesis: A minimally invasive procedure in which the TMJ is flushed with a sterile solution to remove debris and reduce inflammation.

c. Surgery: In rare cases, surgery may be recommended to repair or replace the TMJ joint.

Sleep treatments

Sleep and pain management are intricately connected, with poor sleep often leading to increased pain and chronic pain causing disruptions to sleep. Studies have shown that individuals with chronic pain are more likely to experience poor sleep quality, and individuals with poor sleep quality are more likely to experience chronic pain.

Pain can interfere with sleep by causing discomfort, making it difficult to find a comfortable position, and causing frequent waking. In turn, sleep deprivation can lead to increased pain sensitivity, and can make it difficult for the body to effectively manage and cope with pain.

To address this connection, effective pain management strategies must include addressing sleep quality. This can be done through sleep hygiene practices, such as establishing a regular sleep schedule, creating a relaxing bedtime routine, and minimizing exposure to electronic devices before bedtime.

In addition, behavioral therapies, such as cognitive behavioral therapy for insomnia (CBT-I), can be effective in addressing both sleep and pain. CBT-I helps individuals change negative thought patterns and behaviors that contribute to sleep disturbances, and can help improve sleep quality, reduce pain, and improve overall quality of life.

Medications can also be used to treat sleep disturbances and pain. Sleep aids, such as benzodiazepines or non-benzodiazepine hypnotics, can help individuals fall asleep and stay asleep. Pain relievers, such as nonsteroidal anti-inflammatory drugs (NSAIDs) or opioids, can help reduce pain. However, it is important to use medications only as prescribed, and to discuss the potential risks and benefits with a healthcare provider.

It is important to treat any underlying conditions impacting sleep or quality of sleep. A significant majority of pain patients should undergo a formal sleep study to identify conditions.

An exciting new class of medication includes the Orexin receptor medications. They are a relatively new class of drugs that have shown promise in the treatment of sleep disorders. These medications work by targeting the orexin system in the brain, which is responsible for regulating wakefulness and sleep. By blocking the actions of orexin, these medications can promote sleep and improve sleep quality in people with insomnia and other sleep disorders.

Clinical trials have shown the ability to significantly reduce the time it takes to fall asleep and increase total sleep time. It has also been found to have a favorable safety profile and low risk of dependency or abuse. Examples in this class of medication I use in practice include Dayvigo and Belsomra.

In conclusion, sleep and pain management are interrelated, and addressing one can often have a positive impact on the other. Effective pain management strategies must include addressing sleep quality through sleep hygiene practices, behavioral therapies, and medications, as appropriate. By treating both pain and sleep, individuals can experience improved sleep quality and reduced pain, leading to improved overall quality of life.

Rheumatoid Arthritis

Rheumatoid is a specific condition but there are patient's who are diagnosed with both RA and Fibromyalgia. Rheumatoid arthritis (RA) is a chronic autoimmune disease characterized by inflammation and joint damage. It primarily affects the joints, but it can also affect other organs in the body. RA is a complex condition that requires a multidisciplinary approach for diagnosis and management. In this overview, we will provide a summary of rheumatoid arthritis, including its causes, symptoms, diagnosis, and treatment options.

The exact cause of rheumatoid arthritis remains unknown, but it is believed to result from a combination of genetic and environmental factors. Certain genetic variations and a dysregulated immune response are thought to play a role in triggering the development of RA. Environmental factors such as smoking and certain infections may also contribute to the risk of developing the condition. Women are more commonly affected by RA than men, and the disease typically manifests between the ages of 30 and 50.

RA primarily affects the joints, causing pain, swelling, and stiffness. The joints commonly affected include the hands, wrists, elbows, knees, and feet. The symptoms are often symmetrical, meaning they occur on both sides of the body. In addition to joint involvement, individuals with RA may experience systemic symptoms, such as fatigue, fever, weight loss, and general malaise. Over time, chronic inflammation can lead to joint deformity, reduced range of motion, and functional impairment.

Diagnosing rheumatoid arthritis involves a combination of clinical evaluation, medical history, physical examination, and laboratory tests. The American College of Rheumatology (ACR) criteria are commonly used to aid in the diagnosis. These criteria take into account the number and duration of affected joints, laboratory markers of inflammation, and the presence of rheumatoid factor (RF) and anti-cyclic citrullinated peptide (anti-CCP) antibodies. Imaging techniques such as X-rays, ultrasound, or magnetic resonance imaging (MRI) may also be used to assess joint damage and disease progression.

The treatment of rheumatoid arthritis aims to control symptoms, prevent joint damage, and improve overall quality of life. It typically involves a combination of medications, lifestyle modifications, and supportive therapies. The specific treatment approach may vary depending on the severity of the disease and individual patient factors. Common treatment options include:

1. Disease-Modifying Anti-Rheumatic Drugs (DMARDs): DMARDs, such as methotrexate, sulfasalazine, and hydroxychloroquine, are the cornerstone of RA treatment. These medications help suppress the immune system and reduce inflammation, slowing down joint damage.

2. Biologic Response Modifiers: Biologic DMARDs, including tumor

necrosis factor (TNF) inhibitors, interleukin-6 (IL-6) inhibitors, and other targeted therapies, are prescribed for moderate to severe RA that has not responded to traditional DMARDs. These medications specifically target the molecules involved in the immune response.

3. Nonsteroidal Anti-Inflammatory Drugs (NSAIDs): NSAIDs are used to alleviate pain and reduce inflammation in RA. They provide symptomatic relief but do not alter the disease progression.

4. Corticosteroids: Oral or injected corticosteroids may be prescribed to quickly reduce inflammation and control severe symptoms during disease flares. They are typically used for short-term relief due to potential side effects with long-term use.

5. Physical Therapy and Exercise: Physical therapy can help improve joint mobility, muscle strength, and overall function. Exercise programs tailored to individual needs can help reduce pain and stiffness, as well as improve cardiovascular health and overall well-being.

Lupus

Similar to RA, Lupus is generally diagnosed separate from Fibromyalgia but there are some patients who suffer from both.

Lupus, or systemic lupus erythematosus (SLE), is a chronic autoimmune disease that can affect various organs and systems in the body. It is characterized by inflammation, which occurs when the immune system mistakenly attacks healthy tissues. Lupus can manifest in a wide range of symptoms, including joint pain, skin rashes, fatigue, and organ involvement. While there is no cure for lupus, current treatments aim to manage symptoms, control disease activity, and improve the quality of life for individuals with this condition.

Treatment options for lupus vary depending on the severity and specific manifestations of the disease in each individual. Here is an overview of some of the current treatment approaches:

1. Nonsteroidal Anti-Inflammatory Drugs (NSAIDs): NSAIDs, such as ibuprofen or naproxen, are commonly used to alleviate joint pain, swelling, and stiffness associated with lupus. They provide symptomatic relief but do not target the underlying disease process.

2. Antimalarial Medications: Hydroxychloroquine, a type of antimalarial drug, is often prescribed for lupus due to its

immunomodulatory properties. It can help reduce disease activity, prevent flares, and protect against organ damage. Additionally, hydroxychloroquine has been found to improve skin rashes and joint symptoms in some individuals.

3. Corticosteroids: Corticosteroids, such as prednisone, are potent anti-inflammatory medications used to control severe lupus symptoms or acute flares. They can provide rapid relief but are typically prescribed at the lowest effective dose and for the shortest duration possible due to potential side effects with long-term use.

4. Immunosuppressive Medications: For individuals with more severe or organ-threatening lupus, immunosuppressive drugs may be prescribed. These medications work by suppressing the overactive immune response. Examples include methotrexate, azathioprine, mycophenolate mofetil, and cyclophosphamide. These medications are often used in combination with other treatments to control disease activity and reduce the need for high-dose corticosteroids.

5. Biologic Therapies: In recent years, biologic therapies have emerged as promising options for the treatment of lupus. Belimumab, a monoclonal antibody that targets a specific immune system molecule called B-lymphocyte stimulator (BLyS), has been approved for the treatment of lupus. Other

biologics, such as rituximab and tocilizumab, are sometimes used off-label in refractory cases of lupus.

6. Supportive Therapies: In addition to medical treatments, supportive therapies play a crucial role in managing lupus. Regular monitoring of disease activity and organ involvement, as well as addressing comorbidities such as high blood pressure, osteoporosis, and depression, are important aspects of comprehensive care for individuals with lupus.

It is worth noting that treatment plans for lupus are highly individualized and should be tailored to the specific needs and circumstances of each patient. Close collaboration between the patient, rheumatologist, and other healthcare providers is essential to develop an effective and personalized treatment approach.

OA

Treatment for Osteoarthritis is specifically treated by treated the affected worn down joints or using oral medications to treat OA systemically. For this purpose of our discussion here, we will dive into treatment of Knee Osteoarthritis to give a better example of treating Osteoarthitis.

Knee osteoarthritis (OA) is a common condition in which the protective cartilage in the knee joint breaks down, causing pain, swelling, and stiffness. While knee replacement surgery is often necessary for advanced cases, there are several nonsurgical pain treatments that can help manage symptoms and improve function. These may include:

1. Physical therapy: A physical therapist can work with patients to develop an exercise program that can help strengthen the muscles around the knee joint and improve flexibility and mobility.

2. Weight management: Excess weight can put extra stress on the knee joint, exacerbating symptoms of knee OA. Weight loss through diet and exercise can help alleviate pain and improve function.

3. Medications: Over-the-counter pain relievers such as acetaminophen or nonsteroidal anti-inflammatory drugs (NSAIDs) can help alleviate pain and inflammation associated

with knee OA. Prescription medications, such as corticosteroids or hyaluronic acid injections, may also be used to manage symptoms.

4. Bracing: A knee brace can help provide support and stability to the knee joint, which can alleviate pain and improve function.

5. Topical treatments: Creams, gels, or patches containing capsaicin or menthol may help alleviate pain associated with knee OA.

6. Viscosupplementation has been a very effective treatment for knee OA and deserves it's own chapter.

7. PRP, which will deserve it's own chapter to follow as well.

Viscosupplementation

Viscosupplementation is a nonsurgical treatment option for knee osteoarthritis (OA) that involves injecting a gel-like substance called hyaluronic acid into the knee joint. Hyaluronic acid is a naturally occurring substance in the body that helps lubricate and cushion the joints.

In patients with knee OA, the natural levels of hyaluronic acid in the synovial fluid that surrounds the knee joint are reduced, which can lead to pain and stiffness. Viscosupplementation aims to restore the natural levels of hyaluronic acid in the joint, thereby reducing pain and improving joint function.

The procedure involves injecting the hyaluronic acid gel directly into the knee joint using a needle. The injection is typically performed in a healthcare provider's office and takes only a few minutes. Patients may experience some discomfort during the injection, but this is usually mild and temporary.

The effects of viscosupplementation typically last for six to 12 months and is covered by insurance to be performed every 6 months if necessary. When describing viscosupplementation to patients I like to describe it as "putting WD40 on a squeaky wheel" as we are trying to increase lubrication and to decrease friction/inflammation.

PRP

Platelet-rich plasma (PRP) is a nonsurgical treatment option for knee osteoarthritis (OA) that involves injecting a concentrated solution of a patient's own blood platelets into the affected knee joint. Platelets contain growth factors that can stimulate tissue repair and regeneration.

To prepare PRP, a healthcare provider will draw a small amount of the patient's blood and process it to concentrate the platelets. The resulting PRP solution is then injected into the knee joint using a needle.

PRP injections are typically performed in a healthcare provider's office and take only a few minutes. Patients may experience some discomfort during the injection, but this is usually mild and temporary.

The effects of PRP injections can vary depending on the severity of knee OA and the individual patient. Some patients may experience a reduction in pain and inflammation, as well as improvements in joint function and mobility. The effects of PRP injections may last for several months if not longer. The biggest downside to PRP has been that traditional insurance still views PRP as an 'alternative treatment' and so because of the alternative designation it does fall in to the self pay category of treatment options.

Endometriosis

Endometriosis and fibromyalgia are two separate medical conditions that can coexist in some individuals. Endometriosis is a chronic gynecological disorder characterized by the presence of endometrial-like tissue outside the uterus, commonly causing pain and infertility. Fibromyalgia, on the other hand, is a chronic pain condition characterized by widespread musculoskeletal pain, fatigue, and other associated symptoms. While these conditions have distinct features, they may share some commonalities in terms of treatment approaches and their impact on overall well-being.

The management of endometriosis involves a variety of treatment options depending on the severity of symptoms, the desire for fertility, and individual patient factors. These treatment options include:

1. Pain Medications: Over-the-counter nonsteroidal anti-inflammatory drugs (NSAIDs), such as ibuprofen or naproxen, can help alleviate pain associated with endometriosis. Prescription pain medications may be considered for more severe pain.

2. Hormonal Therapy: Hormonal therapy is commonly used to suppress the growth of endometrial tissue outside the uterus and reduce symptoms. Options include combined oral contraceptives, progestins, gonadotropin-releasing hormone (GnRH) agonists, and danazol.

3. Surgical Interventions: Surgery may be recommended in cases where conservative treatment approaches have not provided sufficient relief. Laparoscopic surgery can be performed to remove endometrial implants, adhesions, and cysts. In severe cases or for those who have completed childbearing, a hysterectomy with removal of both ovaries (total hysterectomy with bilateral salpingo-oophorectomy) may be considered.

4. Assisted Reproductive Technologies (ART): For women with endometriosis-related infertility, in vitro fertilization (IVF) or other ART techniques may be utilized to improve the chances of conception.

CBD and THC

Low-dose THC and CBD oil may be used as part of a comprehensive treatment plan for chronic pain. The exact dosing and formulation will depend on the individual and their specific needs, and it's important to work with a healthcare provider to determine the most appropriate treatment approach.

Here are some current treatment options for chronic pain with low-dose THC and CBD oil:

1. Medical cannabis: In states where medical cannabis is legal, healthcare providers may recommend it as a treatment option for chronic pain. Medical cannabis typically contains both THC and CBD, and the exact ratio of these cannabinoids will vary depending on the strain and formulation.

2. CBD oil: CBD oil is a non-psychoactive cannabinoid that has been shown to have anti-inflammatory and pain-relieving effects. CBD oil is available in various formulations and dosages, and it's important to work with a healthcare provider to determine the most appropriate product and dosing for your specific needs.

3. Low-dose THC/CBD oil: Low-dose THC/CBD oil is a product that contains both THC and CBD in specific ratios. This product may be used as part of a comprehensive treatment plan for chronic pain, and it's important to work with a healthcare

provider to determine the most appropriate formulation and dosing.

4. Topical CBD products: Topical CBD products, such as creams and lotions, can be applied directly to the skin to provide localized pain relief. These products may be particularly useful for joint pain and other types of musculoskeletal pain.

In practice, I have found that the greatest benefit of either low dosed THC or CBD products has been with neuropathic pain and with sleep/anxiety.

I generally do not recommend mixing low dose THC or CBD oil products with traditional narcotics.

Patient Advocacy

As I have stated many times before, fibromyalgia is a complex and often misunderstood condition characterized by chronic pain, fatigue, and a range of other symptoms. Living with fibromyalgia can be challenging, and navigating the healthcare system to receive appropriate care can be overwhelming. This is where patient advocacy plays a crucial role. Patient advocacy involves actively seeking information, understanding one's rights, and effectively communicating with healthcare providers to ensure the best possible care. Additionally, joining advocacy groups allows individuals with fibromyalgia to come together, share experiences, and collectively work towards raising awareness and improving the understanding of this condition. In this discussion, we will explore the importance of patient advocacy in treating fibromyalgia, both as an individual being their own advocate and as a member of advocacy groups.

Being Your Own Advocate:

1. Education and Knowledge: As a patient with fibromyalgia, it is essential to educate yourself about the condition. Understanding the symptoms, treatment options, and available resources empowers you to make informed decisions about your care. Stay up-to-date with current research and treatment advancements to have meaningful conversations with healthcare providers.

2. Effective Communication: Effective communication with healthcare providers is key to ensuring that your concerns and needs are heard. Clearly articulate your symptoms, express your treatment goals, and ask questions to fully understand your diagnosis and treatment plan. Actively engage in discussions about treatment options, including medications, lifestyle modifications, and alternative therapies.

3. Building a Supportive Healthcare Team: Building a supportive healthcare team is crucial in managing fibromyalgia. Seek out healthcare providers who are knowledgeable about fibromyalgia and who listen to your concerns. Collaborate with them to develop a personalized treatment plan that takes into account your specific needs and goals.

4. Tracking Symptoms and Treatment: Keep a symptom journal to track your fibromyalgia symptoms, their severity, and any triggers or patterns you notice. This information can help you and your healthcare team identify effective treatment strategies and make informed decisions about your care.

Joining Advocacy Groups:

1. Community and Support: Joining advocacy groups provides an opportunity to connect with others who understand the challenges of living with fibromyalgia. Sharing experiences,

knowledge, and coping strategies can provide a sense of community and support. Online forums, support groups, and social media platforms dedicated to fibromyalgia can be valuable resources for connecting with others.

2. Raising Awareness: Advocacy groups play a vital role in raising awareness about fibromyalgia among the general public, healthcare professionals, and policymakers. By sharing personal stories, participating in awareness campaigns, and organizing events, advocacy groups help dispel misconceptions and promote a better understanding of fibromyalgia.

3. Influencing Research and Policy: Advocacy groups can actively participate in research initiatives, clinical trials, and policy discussions related to fibromyalgia. By engaging in these activities, they can contribute to the development of new treatment options, improved healthcare policies, and increased funding for research.

4. Access to Resources: Advocacy groups often provide access to educational materials, resources, and expert advice on managing fibromyalgia. They can help connect individuals with reputable healthcare providers, research studies, support groups, and other valuable resources.

In Conclusion, patient advocacy plays a critical role in effectively managing fibromyalgia. Being your own advocate empowers you to actively participate in your treatment decisions, communicate effectively with healthcare providers, and seek the best possible care. Joining advocacy groups allows individuals to connect with others, share experiences, raise awareness, and influence research and policy initiatives. I would like to give a special shout out to the Support Fibromyalgia Network, @beingfibromom on instagram and @painmgmt_md on tiktok for their advocacy work. By being proactive and engaged, individuals with fibromyalgia can have a significant impact on their own well-being and the broader fibromyalgia community.

Congrats Fibro PainWarrior!

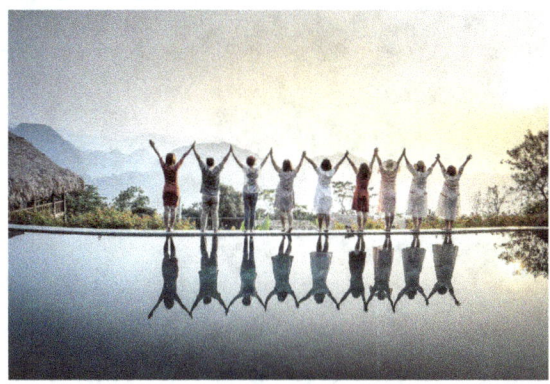

I want to send a congratulations to anyone who took the time to make it through my entire Patient's Guide to Fibromyalgia. I hope you have found some useful information and have come to realize that their is hope for treating your fibromyalgia pain. I truly believe that every patient with fibromyalgia can find a decreased level of pain and improved level of function. As this book details, it takes you being an active participant in your treatment. Find yourself a local multidisciplinary team to help you on your journey. I hope my insights from my past 23 years of practice have given you some actionable information to discuss with your local healthcare providers. For taking on this journey you are no longer merely a patient instead you are a warrior, a Fibro PainWarrior. You will continue to battle and not give in to the pain. I am confident you will find peace and success along your journey!

About the Author

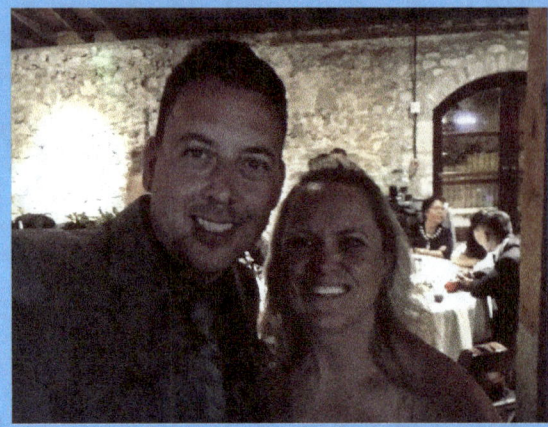

Matthew Dovie is also the author of The Patient's Guide to Pain Management. Matthew Dovie has 23 years of experience as a head APP within interventional pain management.

Matthew Dovie has also gained social media success with @painmgmt_md on tiktok that at the time of publishing has over 30,000 followers and over 4 million views.